Love, Miracles and Medicine Men

Adventures with an Indigenous Healer

Mary Ruehl-Keiser

Writers Club Press

San Jose New York Lincoln Shanghai

Love, Miracles and Medicine Men
Adventures with an Indigenous Healer

Published by Writers Club Press
an imprint of iUniverse.com, Inc.

For information address:
iUniverse.com, Inc.
620 North 48th Street
Suite 201
Lincoln, NE 68504-3467
www.iuniverse.com

ISBN: 0-595-00973-5

Printed in the United States of America

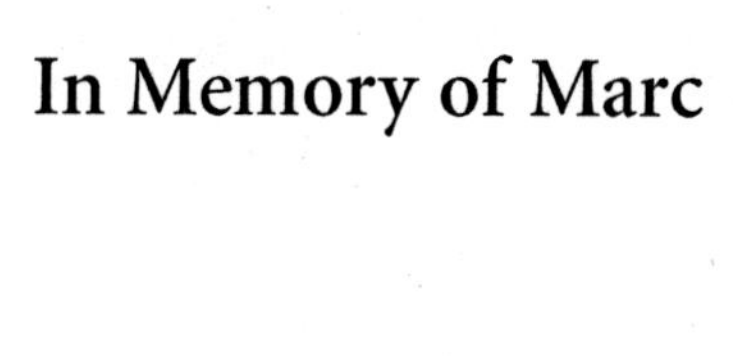
In Memory of Marc

Epigraph

The medicine man turns a mental image into a physical reality-in fact, this is what all miracle workers do. At the quantum level they "see" a new result, and in that vision the new result emerges.

Deepak Chopra—How to Know God
Learning is finding out what you already know.
Doing is demonstrating that you know it
Teaching is reminding others that they know just as well as you.
You are all learners, doers, teachers

Richard Bach—Illusions

Foreword

How can I ever begin to explain a story such as this. No, it's not fiction, but reads like one. No, we are not completely crazy, in fact, Jann and I both hold responsible jobs in our 'other world' back in Illinois. This is not a story where I hope to convince you to support a new guru or join a cult. It is simply a story that weaves through two distinct cultures which carry two distinct avenues of healing that come clashing together, oftentimes creating chaos and confusion, but eventually ending with mutual respect for each others' values and beliefs.

After reading this tale, do I want you to hop in the car and head toward South Dakota? Do I think all standard medical practices should cease and be replaced with indigenous healing? Would I want you to cast aside your beliefs and values, for the sake of mine? Hardly. But, I would ask for two things—tolerance and an open mind. Why and how I was lead to the heart of Native Americans, I'm not sure, but I know it was a long, slow process that took over two decades of self exploration, spiritual dark nights of the soul, and trekking down multiple dead end streets of new age philosophy. My one salvation was having a friend to share in these ups and downs. Her name is Jann.

She and I work in the health care profession as nurses. Her specialty is critical care nursing, while mine floats between quality assessment and hospice. Who knows why the winds of restlessness move through a person, thought to be content in their unchanging, upper middle class world and blows them into strange lands where odd meets bizarre. We, unlike Dorothy, asked to ride the tornado and be transported to Oz. And we were! Perhaps since both of us dealt heavily in life/death situations we were thrust into afterlife and other life explorations. We often found we had too many questions and not enough answers, but the most puzzling question was—Why aren't others asking the same thing? Step by step we found answers to some of them. Never will all the mysteries be solved, for that is the challenge of life and the demands of faith.

Jann and I had many comical experiences-some self created and others self inflicted by Native friends. She and I discovered one truth through our longtime quest. If we discovered humor in our teachers, as well as the ability to laugh at ourselves and take a slightly lighter approach to heavy issues—it was a good path. If you are academia inclined and wish credible documentation backed by reputable bibliographies, or your mind runs in a scientific vein and demands factual evidence validated by blind studies and medical data to credit shaman healing then close the book now! This is a simple story, entwined with light hearted humor that relays a story as deep and old as time itself—Man's search for meaning and purpose and his relationship to the Great Mystery.

Charles. How can I briefly sum up a well fitting description of a man who still blows me away with his connection to the 'powers', has the innocence of a prankster child, the ego of a man, and never ending dedication and commitment to follow his spiritual path. He is no 'holy man', as he puts it. He doesn't wish for you to drop everything and follow him. He wants to be known as one thing—a human being. And the main focus of his journey through life is finding other human beings. He at times chastises my distinction of the red and white race and tells me to label it one way. Human Beings! There is no separation.

He and his wife Hazel are well known in producing traditional Native American art work. Their days are filled with work, as well as fostering children at home, not to mention the constant stream of people who show up at his door to be taught or healed. The true calling of a Shaman is not an easy road.

Respect! For all living things is probably the key focus in Native American Spirituality. Honoring and truly believing we are all connected through one loving presence of Spirit is the crux of their culture. Discovering, on our own, these two simple philosophies has made a profound effect on our lives that burns deep into our souls. We couldn't ask for anything more except to share our story with others.

In the words of Albert Einstein:

A human being is part of the whole called by us "Universe," a part limited in time and space. He experiences himself, his thoughts and feelings, as something separated from the rest, a kind of optical delusion of his consciousness. This delusion is a kind of prison for us, restricting us to our personal desires and to affection for a few persons nearest us. Our task must be to free ourselves from this prison by widening our circle of compassion to embrace all living creatures and the whole nature in its beauty.

In the words of Lakota:
MITKUYE OYASIN
"We are all related"

Acknowledgements

When I first met Charles he offered to fix my eyes. I gave him one of my 'head thick as a brick' looks since I felt, aside from these middle age eyes needing readers, they were just fine. I heard Charles say he would work on my eyes. The word he actually used was vision and between those two simple words lies and expansive canyon of interpretation. It is here I wish to thank and acknowledge his wonderful positive presence in my life and bless him for at last restoring my 'vision.'

A special thanks and recognition to my dear friend Jann (Two Knives) who without her wit, dedication to helping mankind, and unquenchable thirst for self fulfillment this book would not have been written. Through our many wild and oftentimes mis-adventures, her ceaseless giving nature brought love and laughter to those who came in contact with her. Jann's sense of humor was the instrumental key that opened the door to the Lakota heart.

Introduction

ONCE UPON A TIME, IN THE BLACK HILLS OF SOUTH DAKOTA…

It was midnight and my daughter Kate had just eased into her sleeping bag on the living room floor of a Native American's home when suddenly she sensed something in the kitchen doorway staring at her. The hairs on the back of her neck immediately stood up at attention. She turned cautiously and looked up. Nothing! Just an over active imagination, she thought, conceived from ghostly tales attached to this place. Kate rolled over with her back toward the kitchen and forced herself to take a slow deep breath. She lay there waiting, stiff as a wooden log, all neuron fibers on alert and waiting.

The sensation came again, like a dark cloud hovering, causing her to catapult into an upright position and peer cautiously into the black unlit room. Again she was greeted by nothing. The only audible sound she heard was the occasional drip of a leaky sink faucet as it kept time to ordinary reality. Relief swept over her, like a tidal wave, pushing her back to the shores of common sense. The faucet continued its serenade as well as an occasional snore from the back bedrooms and within moments she was convinced her imagination had been working overtime. The other young women remained sleeping by her side, leaving Kate even more isolated as she gazed at their soft slumbering faces.

She became aware of the rain pelting against the roof outside and gave a sigh of relief; grateful she was not out there. Thunder rumbled nonstop in the distance. 'Great scene for a horror flick', she thought while attempting to rub the goose bumps from her flesh. Why had she listened to those dull-witted spooky stories about spirits roaming this place?

Suddenly, the presence was back. Kate sensed a penetrating stare boring holes through the back of her head. This time, it was so strong she felt she could reach out and touch it. She turned quickly and looked. Blackness. 'That's it', she thought, her heart thumping erratically in her chest, 'now I can't even sleep inside the house.'

Then came the growl! The first time it was a low snarling, menacing sound. She reasoned it was Charles, the Medicine Man who owned the house, up to his antics. But how did he sneak into the kitchen? Both entryways were within her range of vision and hearing. She was also aware of the fact that when Charles placed people up on the mountain for Vision Quests, he became more somber and serious. There were two on the hill that night, in the midst of the thunderstorm. One was her mother and now she wondered about her safety.

'NO!' Kate reasoned. 'Stay within the walls of logic.' She was there to support her mother, which meant she must be strong. She lay there, refusing to accept any answer but the most rational. Unfortunately the logical was beginning to pale.

The growl came again, this time roaring enough to awaken and terrify the others who lay next to her. Chaos ensued as eyes opened wide. The only noise now heard was the loud swishing sound of nylon, as people flew out of their sleeping bags, groping for each others hands in the dark and hoarsely whispering: "What the hell was that?"

In the next instant the entire kitchen illuminated in a flash of white light, unlike any form of lightening. The three panicked women made frantic grasps for the light switch. What makes a sound such as that? A bear? A wolf? Some other massive sized predatory beast? In the house? And the light, like nothing ever seen before, but what?

Then it was gone. As quick as it came—the light, the noise—the only evidence of disturbance were three stunned woman left huddled on the floor. They sat there frozen, hearts pounding wildly, trying to organize their fragmented thoughts. Kate clicked on the TV and living room lamps, hoping any further noise or disturbance would be blamed on the tube or openly seen. Eventually, all of the young women lay back down quiet—but waiting.

It would be another long sleepless night at the home of the Medicine Man. A first time experience for Kate and the other young women, however, now with hairs standing on end and goose bumps the size of Easter eggs, Kate safely reasoned it may be her last. She remembered her mother's tall tales from earlier summers and had teasingly replied that perhaps mom and her friend were exaggerating a bit?

All the stories her mother told could be explained, she felt, mainly by Charles playing games, or so one would think. But now, here she was on the living room floor, instead of out in her tent, because it was too 'spooky' out there and now too 'spooky' in here.

Kate mentally recalled a camping trip last year, to the bottom of the Grand Canyon, where wild cats had boldly jumped across their sleeping cots while they slept. 'That,' she now thought, 'was a mild fright compared to this.' What goes on here can't be reasoned away by simple logic. Instead, it is a place where childhood fears and unfinished lessons resurface in dark corners to taunt and teach, but this time there are no mothers or logical explanations to fade them into fantasy.

How could she tell others about these tales? Who would believe? She hardly could herself. But they did happen. Didn't they?

Chapter One

As I write this down, I think of all the people who will read these pages and be assured that I am dancing on the edge of sanity. This is not a logical composition created for the white western mentality, nor is it meant to support new age fluff. It is simply a story of a white woman (actually two of us) and their search for truth in a world encased in teasing deceptions.

I am grateful my daughter Kate also bears witness to such events and helps deflect some caustic remarks that question my good mental health from family members and friends. Kate's first intention, I'm sure, was to discover a new path and culture as a spectator. Now, her present day beliefs have altered radically and her new Native American friends are held in high regard, not to mention complete respect for their spiritual practice.

The first reasonable question that should be laid on the table is: What brings one to the door of a Lakota Medicine Man, where time stands still, reality sprouts from an entirely different direction, and life takes on a whole new meaning?

We are talking first and foremost about two women who were born and bred from the white lily ponds of the Midwest and who believed that things of nature where contained in a zoo, sweating was socially unacceptable and Indians were in history books and, according to the Catholic version, killed a lot of Jesuits.

I sprouted from a family that subjectively hinted their prejudices. We were not raised to hate or dislike anyone, but neither did we socialize with or discuss those other races. In my teens, I was hardly enlightened to anyone's plights as hormones kicked in and over ruled any and all forms of social consciousness. My main path led right to the opposite sex and my environment was so white I needed sunglasses to lesson the glare. It is not my intention to lay blame on upbringing for in the early decades of my life I held as much intellectual and emotional depth as a thin crust pizza. I was raised with strong family values, a very happy childhood compared to most. Later, in the course of my parochial education, I was pulverized and molded by nuns insuring a deep seeded faith—One that would mentally taunt me with guilt and fear at the beginning of the search for MY truth.

My partner and friend on this spiritual sojourn is Jann, who on the other hand was slightly more liberal. In her youth she took on the causes of several politically incorrect injustices. Jann has always danced to the beat of a different drummer and the Native Americans love her beat.

Although we had shared new age quests over the past several years she, nor I, were hardly prepared to camp out in the yard of a Medicine Man every summer and accept as reality all the events that occurred there. We were nurses employed at a community hospital in an upper class neighborhood whose only claim to Native American sympathy was viewing Dances with Wolves and stating they liked it.

Some years back, Jann had received a life altering wake up call when taking a seminar with a Comanche Medicine Man in Tucson. This man, Edgar, was well known in the circle of hospital health care professionals. Jann, also a nurse, was drawn to the seminar. After a week of intense ceremony and deep self-exploration, not to mention multiple boxes of tissue, she came back with an opened heart and eager mind pushing to know more about these people.

She remembers one sizzling summer day in 1990, when she was given the name of a spiritual guide, as she lazily drifted across her pool deep in meditation and sun tan oil. He called himself Red Cloud. She laughed at the name and thought it must be the cousin to White Cloud bathroom tissue. She suspected she was a prime source of entertainment in the spirit realm. She could hardly imagine at that moment how fate would take her to the land of Red Cloud a few years down the road.

We plowed through many alternative and non traditional healing adventures as the health profession was our mainstay in life. When first exploring the indigenous path we were often left breathless and exhausted trying to balance what is real vs. unreal while attempting to make sense of their world. Those things that commit people in our white world to institutions are considered honorable and valid testimony of the Great Mystery's presence in their lives.

The first time I heard Charles, our Lakota Medicine man, talk I was absolutely clue-less. My main concern was: Where are the silver braids and aged face? I expected all medicine men to be very wise old sages.

Yet, there he stood in his early fifties, a man already instrumental in curing cancer some fifteen years back. It was knowledge of that cure, directly from the man who was healed, which eventually brought me to the Black Hills.

Often times, one needs to have experienced pain in their lives to spark a new direction and challenge one's old forms of belief. I attended a lecture on the Native American pipe back in the early nineties. The man giving the lecture stated he developed kidney cancer in the nineteen seventies and had been healed by a Native American shaman. I had recently lost a young brother to the same cancer and was thunderstruck, not to mention filled with regret, that I had not discovered this man or method sooner.

I had instigated several alternative-healing techniques with my younger brother during his illness and when our little support group would gather to meditate with him, my intuitive sister in law would comment that a spirit she called Cochise, was sitting in the corner. This is the point where one needs to be open and understand how many people do sense other then normal reality occurrences when someone you love hangs on the fringe of life. We were hardly a family of fantasy or fortunetellers.

Yet, when worlds get turned upside down and hope becomes quite scarce, other senses come in to play. People grasp, like children on the merry go round, for the brass ring of optimism. No one willing to let go and fall into the belief that all that can be done, has been. But it did end with his death, throwing all who loved him into a tailspin of depression, and like most family members, we asked what more we could have done. I had come to terms with the acceptable answer.

Everything that could be done, was done. End of story.

Now, as I sat and listened to this man, three years later, all I could think about was—Why didn't I pay more attention to that something in the corner? This man's lecture on the Indigenous world was the initial bait on the hook as I had recently developed a keen interest in Native American History—especially the Lakota.

Sitting Bull is one of my favorite historical characters. The healed man who stood before us claimed to possess one of Sitting Bull's pipes. The pipe brought me to his lecture. The story about his cure eventually brought me to Charles.

Lakotas who had more or less embraced him for his dedication and assistance in reclaiming their artifacts gave the pipe to him. The man, some years later, was stricken with kidney cancer. Charles, a Lakota Medicine Man was asked to stop by and see this adopted member of their tribe as he suffered in the final throes of cancer.

Charles, along with his brother, entered the hospital late one night and quietly walked up to the Cancer Ward asking to see their very sick friend. They were given permission due to the man's moribund condition. Charles then asked if he could smoke his pipe. The staff was indignant at the thought of someone asking to smoke on this terminal unit, until Charles explained that a Pipe is the sacred messenger for the Lakota and part of the healing ceremony. After entering the dying man's room, Charles lit the pipe and prayed with his brother and when his prayers were finished casually commented—"You really have it bad. It will take about four days to go away."

In four days, the man was feeling better, his blood work came swiftly back to baseline, the doctors were at a loss for words. That was twenty years ago. The man is now married with a young child, all previous signs of the illness vanished.

The healed storyteller now passed Sitting Bull's pipe around for each of us to pray. At that time, I wasn't sure to whom I was praying. All I could feel was confusion by this Great Mystery God of theirs. My reasoning, at a child's level, began to feel betrayed by the god that took my brother while this god seemed to heal. I was a nurse and Christian—soon both would appear insignificant in this strange and foreign world.

Chapter Two

Jann and I became fast friends in the early nineties. Perhaps I caught sight of a medicine bag, or crystal dangling from her otherwise conservative ICU scrubs and felt a connection. Together, we ventured down several new age and transpersonal lanes, at last both settling into native wannabees. Everywhere we went, our attire became more native. Needless to say, we hardly looked inconspicuous in a large mid western city sporting deerskin and feathers.

We often found ourselves with people of questionable sanity, making this road much more adventuresome than daily patient charting. We found our path veering into parts unknown, like 'trekkies', often seated inside lean-tos in desolate environments, holding very odd conversations with very odd people.

Each time we drove up some deserted looking driveway and were greeted by some wild eyed looking person in the hopes of learning new healing alternative techniques, I would quiver and beg to leave the scene, as I was convinced death was imminent.

Jann always reassuring me that we would make it out alive. I'm not sure how she knew that.

In the beginning, our spiritual search was scattered to the winds as we meditated with Buddhists monks, became pretzels with a Yogi, learned to re-breathe through our hurts, and new-breathe into bliss. Carl Jung became our mentor and Wayne Dyer, our savior. We danced with Sufi's and became more than Christ Conscious, but the Natives still held first place in our hearts. The pull to go west became overpowering.

1995 was the first time I ventured to South Dakota. My husband and I traveled through the Black Hills as typical tourists while Jann was already camped out that summer at the Medicine Man's house with her friends. Her friends had come to know Charles over the past couple years through their professor friend—the same man I had listened to while holding Sitting Bull's pipe. I am always amazed by these acts of synchronicity. Needless to say, I was more than eager to visit with Charles and eventually we connected with the group at the Crazy Horse Memorial Restaurant.

Truly, some of the oddest people to date were seen at this Restaurant as they sprinkled in through the doors decorated like a cross between Custer's last stand and the Ben Franklin five and ten. Heads were shaved and ears decorated with multiple dangling earrings and feathers. You could definitely identify the Native Americans. They were the ones dressed simply in T-shirts, jeans and gym shoes. I could sense the spiritual cocktail party about to begin.

My husband could not remove the dumbfounded expression from his face. He began shifting in his seat, a sign the flight or fight hormone had kicked in.

There were gaggles of people surrounding Charles that night, making it impossible to get close. Jann sat next to me during dinner, bubbling with enthusiasm and slightly spooked by several ghostly stories fondly conveyed by her newfound Native friends. Even the children discovered fun in teasing her about all the spirits hovering around the house. She wasn't sure if she should believe or bolt.

I was invited back to his house that night. At last I would meet *The Man*. My husband, finding some of the experience a little unsettling for his German Catholic upbringing, politely declined the invitation and was dropped back at the lodge.

Jann escorted me to Charles house, repeating all recent conversations along the way. My ears were at full attention as we drove through the Black Hills. I could not wait to get there. When it came to the topic of

Christianity, I was somewhat taken aback as I listened to her stories. Some of Charles beliefs appeared to be quoted right from a novel I was developing. I kept asking Jann if she told him about my book. She denied any giving away of my secret story and I knew she had limited information about its contents. Odd, I thought and decided I would have to mention that to Charles. So, there I was, one late night five years ago, walking up his front porch steps in South Dakota, unaware my life would soon steer in a new direction.

I noticed several people sitting out on the deck but the chair next to Charles was empty. He motioned for me to sit next to him. I should have known right then the cosmic set up was in first gear.

He continued to talk with his guests, my presence hardly interrupting his thoughts, and as my heart slowed back to normal beat , for I am always fearful of unknown adventures, I began to listen to his words and soon discovered that the person he was presently describing to them was myself. He had somehow unzipped my persona, right before my eyes, and reached in and read my soul. I felt myself slowly glissade down the chair and shift positions several times, searching for a small black hole to fall into. I hardly felt comfortable!

By the looks in others eyes they hardly seemed aware of what he was doing, or perhaps were just being polite as they also had once occupied the hot seat. He never directed his eyes or words to me, but we both knew. Instead he would say: "Some people are like this..." and my worst flaw would come hurtling at me, like a cracked raw egg, ready to splatter in my face. At one point, the topic arose regarding how people grieve and are unwilling to let go. He talked about ongoing grief, as if it were a high offense, and clenched his fists to exemplify its detriments to both the living and the spirits. Those pitiful mourners left behind would often become ill themselves, he said while sadly shaking his head. Because they refuse to move forward and let go of the pain.

"Some people grieve for three years, some for five, and some" as he turned to me for the first time with eye contact, " hang on for eight years!" My brother had been dead exactly eight years that summer. I got the message.

He then moved on to tell me his version of Christianity. I was astounded to hear the tale run similar to the fiction story I was creating and mentioned, in a light fashion, we must be tuned into the same wavelength. He seemed to ignore my comment. Obviously, I was not impressing this man with my wit.

When at times he gave me eye contact I felt I was peering into some wise old sage's eyes instead of the character next to me in black denim and gym shoes. He seems to transform into this ancient power. The topic then moved on to the significance and importance of the Purification Ceremony—the Sweat. He somehow knew my sheer terror of the sweat lodge experience and later that evening led me down to his and gently coaxed me in to look around while it lay stone cold.

"Next time you come," he said, "you will do a sweat and return to the womb." I had doubted there would be a next time and besides I had just completed hyper-ventilating breath work, back in Chicago, to get re-birthed out of the womb.

At times he could be endearing and nurturing while other times he cut to the quick, but he was gentle with me on our first meeting, realizing my fearful nature.

When I rose to leave his black piercing eyes looked long and hard at me and he asked-"Now are you going to write that book?" (So, he had heard me, after all.) His voice grew louder as he repeated the question and suddenly the winds picked up. The trees then started to creak and bend with enough ruckus that people inside the house came out to see. (My analytical mind raced into overtime and asked—how did he time that question to the wind?) Charles locked into my eyes and said: "Why do you think I was telling that story?

I knew you were coming and I told others that tale so you would believe! Now, are you going to write that book even if it means you will not be liked or people will get angry with you?" (The trees seemed bent in half by this point)

I'm sure my face showed utter confusion as I lip-synched the word—"YES!" The winds ceased. For the next few moments everyone just stood around in silence trying to collect their thoughts. I came home and told that story to many and thought about him and his people for the entire year and knew, without a doubt, I would return.

The following year, Jann and I jumped into a rented car and headed west to the Black Hills. We had mixed feelings as to whether this was the correct path for us to be following. Somehow our idea of a master, guru or spiritual advisor was a little softer than Charles. His looks were as piercing as the hawk at times and we could not help but feel like prey. I knew the cruelties bestowed on his people by the whites were not that far back in his ancestral lines, and I thought: *What if this is the ultimate pay back—to fool these dumb white people into running scared?*

As we sped toward South Dakota the road was an endless ribbon through flat unchanging scenery that left Jann and I bored senseless. It wasn't long before we began ranting and raving about our personal lives, to pass the time. We both took a high dive into the pity pot gathering all recent complaints toward our lives and spilling them out, but not forgetting to chomp on the last of our sandwiches as we did. Finally we came into Rapid City, our marathon trip coming to a close, so we thought. We had driven eight hundred and fifty three miles, now all we needed was a friendly greeting and rest. Instead, we took a wrong turn and were lost at the last stretch of our trip, stirring more irritation into our stewing personalities. We saw Mt. Rushmore from every possible view as we passed it about 8 times. As the sun started to set, I could feel Jann fidgeting in her seat. She was beginning to recall the ghost stories of last year. Finally after a few phone calls and a Native American risking his life to flag us down as we sped by him at seventy miles an hour, we arrived up the driveway just in time to be urgently greeted and rushed into a Sweat Ceremony.

The mental preparation for a sweat had taken me one full year of coming to terms with. We, two nurses, could not reasonably explain why a person doesn't succumb to death in there. Jann had experienced his sweat lodge the year before. All she could say is she prayed for death! That did not leave me feeling at ease. She was convinced we could bring in a few raw chickens, corn and potatoes and have a prepared meal when over. The final thought was—if it's that hot, why aren't my muscles cooking?

I had compromised with the left side of my brain to possibly tolerate one sweat and perhaps that one would be at the end of the trip. And, certainly I would not act foolish and attempt to make it through the entire four doors, which lasts approximately three hours.

Now, here we are, stomachs loaded to the max, tempers flying, suffering from near exhaustion and I'm being cajoled by the Medicine Man as he imitates clacking chicken sounds in response to my excuses. Jann and I look at each other and caught the resignation in each other's eyes. In complete surrender we marched up to the house to change clothes. At last we entered the sweat lodge, feeling like we had held up the party from the looks on the other sweat lodge guests. I was convinced my life was over, even caught a few last minute flashbacks and as I crawl into the lodge I am placed between two Native American women, older than I with huge grinning smiles, looking like they were ready to embark on a cruise ship instead of a hot trip to hell. At this point my heart was racing. I did not think hearts could pound as wildly and remain inside one's chest. I was convinced I was about to die and it would be between two smiling Indians.

But being the fearful human creature I am and completely exhausted by constant battle, I had decided it was time to face my fears and if it required dying—then just do it and be quiet about it! I crawled into his sweat that year, convinced it was the end. All I needed was the white light and tunnel. The atmosphere was already stifling and the hot rocks had not been brought in yet. He sat there for several minutes, before beginning the ceremony and sternly looked across the lodge at Jann and myself. We awaited his words of wisdom; instead he began repeating—word for word—all of our complaints spilled to each other in our final hours drive along I-90. He admonished us for acting like victims and complained of seeing two children instead of women across from him. And through all this the women on either side of me continued their smiles and soft prayers.

Before going further, I might add that these reprimands are not meant to belittle another human, in fact they are, I feel, not even coming from Charles a great deal of the time. It is another force that moves through him and looks through his eyes as he lays out your petty complaints. Jann and I looked at each other in astonishment, wondering how he could know all this.

And, my how that man loves a hot sweat! We made it through two doors that day, grateful we could still remember who we were when it was over. Jann had mentioned she thought he must have some kind of cigarette lighter in there as these little zipping noises and small flashes of light appear. I eventually rationalized it must be some form of heat lighting phenomena. Ha! One has to appreciate the Native American Sweat in person.

There are no words to describe, at first the fear, then the sacredness of this ceremony. When it began, I listened to his Lakota Prayers and the drumming with half ears and heart for my fear was overpowering me. I could not see in front of my eyes, as only black enveloped us. But eventually, my heartbeat fell into synch, with every beat of the drum, followed by a mind at last willing to settle down. All the fellow sweat lodge participants were singing and their melody quickly swept me up, pulling me into the experience and its mystery. Soon, I felt it an honor to be witnessing, no partaking, in such an event. But still that left side of my brain, scolding me for how unchristian this all is.

What I came to understand is how pre-Christian it all is. Not something added after the missionaries' attempts to pollute or abolish their religion, but still a strong moving force that remained the same for millenniums. Native American spirituality alive and well after so many centuries of abuse and intolerance, with its people through time enduring severe punishments to insure its survival. Their courage and determination overwhelms me. Several of the old cultures had similar nature related rituals, before they too were condemned and obliterated from the earth and replaced with fear of demons and ancient ceremonies, such as this one, labeled evil and pagan.

I heard different prayers that day; just as honorable and sincere as the ones I had been taught. We laughed (barely) in between the doors, which allow a short reprieve from the heat. We shared sips of cool water from the same ladle passed around the lodge and I never considered how many germs could be passed along with it. I learned when it became too hot at times to remain sitting up, to lie upon the cool damp earth and place my cheek on her for comfort and not worry if my face was muddy.

There are no words that can describe crawling out of that lodge late at night and lying on the damp ground, watching steam rise from your body and looking up at those millions of stars, with a group of former strangers now feeling like one, not only with them but all of your surroundings, and I wonder how I ever existed without this. I have never felt prayers move through me before like they do in the lodge. Nor, have I sensed someone listen to my prayers like I know they are listening in there and even the zipping noises and heat lightening flashes never danced around a man made altar in a Church I have attended, as it does in that small adobe shaped hut, that can cook chickens, heal people and drive away man made fears in one fell swoop!

And back home the family and friends first question—Why in God's name would you do that? And in simple reply—it seems to me the only place I find God and hear His name!!

Did you know that Stars dance in the sky? Laying on the grass one night, after a sweat in South Dakota, I was directed to look at some of them, as they seem to jump and leap around. Of course I rubbed my eyes several times, insisting, like you are right now, that there is some logical and scientific explanation for this visualization. But there wasn't and they just do!

Chapter Three

I have a quirky little mind with an over active imagination and a husband that believes the word emotional is perhaps a four letter profanity. His fondness for pets holds steadfast to this belief—unless they are useful or edible, they have no place in his life. If I lived alone I would probably be in one of those condemned houses you read about with multitudes of four legged creatures scurrying about the place. My favorites are cats, preferably tigers. Second place ranks the wolf. My attraction to predatory beings probably is a statement about my personality. My husband has lived that truth.

But the one animal that did seem to mesmerize my spouse was the buffalo. He sat for hours staring out his car window at these massive beasts in Custer Park, South Dakota. I found them less then attractive, but seeing them this close left me to wonder how the Native Americans survived the hunts against these fearsome giants and were not driven into extinction. It is hard to believe arrows penetrated that thick hide of theirs.

Bison are aggressive, as some tourists discovered when attempting to video them out of the car. They move for no one. My husband, so taken by them, was even generous enough to offer me a hide one year for my birthday. But, knowing it would never blend appropriately in a suburbia home, I opted for a computer instead.

In Custer, we gazed at the mammoth creature from a distance but at different points in time I came to meet him face to face. My husband and I took another vacation the following year, to the shores of Lake Erie in Ohio, and behold, they had a Safari Land. In this hidden land of adventure, located behind a Wal-Mart Super Store, the only truly African creatures we witnessed were zebras and giraffes, the rest were a smattering from every other country. Guests were invited to feed these charming animals through open windows with plastic containers filled with dry pellet food. I was aghast at the thought of leaving the windows down? But nature always calls to me and how often does one get to pet zebras and giraffes?

We traveled down the road as each beast jammed his head inside the window to greedily grab for the food. My mother sat in the back with a huge grin and windows rolled up. I began to feel at ease after the giraffe finally pulled his head out of our car along with his twelve inches tongue and the zebra finally stopped chewing on our steering wheel. And feeling right with the world, I gazed back to my window only to be greeted with piles of knotty brown fur tickling my nose. Before we could roll up my window, an immense buffalo attempted to push his head into my lap. At first I was concerned as they were less than friendly at Custer Park, but this Ohio relation felt obvious affection for the plastic bowl filled with pellets sitting on my lap. Enough to jam his head inside the car and press his full weight into my breasts.

My husband, repulsed by a wild creature slobbering all over his Cadillac cried: “Get the buffalo out of the car!!” He did not appear as impressed with them as in Custer Park.

With futile attempts, I shoved against the buffalo’s forehead, then in his mouth, finally against his nose, all the while so weak from laughter at my husband’s ridiculous petition to move this half-ton beast off my body that the creature only advanced more in the car then out.

Finally bored by the lack of pellets, he pulled away but not before he gave one snort that filled the car with such a noxious odor that we almost fell over from the fumes. The animal gave full meaning to the term buffalo breath! When the mighty bison at last squeezed back out the window, there, waiting patiently behind him was his best pal the

Long Horn. My horrified husband desperately reached for the window controls while envisioning the roof lining in his car shredded to bits.

I left safari land with full respect for a culture, which spent its life on the plains hunting mammoth creatures such as this, while we presently find it inconvenient to run out to the kitchen to prepare an instant dinner. Since placing my hands all over that creatures face and being that up close and personal with him, I have since grown fond of the Buffalo and use him as a symbol of endurance.

During winter storms in the great plains, this enormous beast always faced his head into the blizzard and each time there is an uprising in my life, I think of that creature out on the land, standing there staunchly enduring, and hope for the courage to face my storms and hold steadfast.

History taught us our predecessors killed these animals for fifty cents on the hide, but the slaughter was also done with the underlying intention to starve out the tribes that relied on their meat. When placing my hands on the buffalo's head and staring into those big brown, vacant eyes I was thankful he was still here. Just like their two legged counterparts, the Native Americans, these mammoth creatures barely survived the white man's invasion.

Now, since the wolf is my favorite American animal, I actually sought out a connection to getting a part wolf puppy (enough wolf to satisfy me). But, if I brought it into my home with my not nature loving mate, the pup and I would both be out on the street before saying I'll blow your house down. So, to appease myself I imagined what it would be like to have my very own pet wolf.

Of course, I realize it would be cruel to contain such a beautiful beast and attempt to domesticate it, however, this is MY imagination and I can redesign all rules and ethics and make my wolf very happy to live inside my house. My imaginary wolf was a she and I envisioned her quite large with a heavy grayish coat and beautiful eyes. At night I would picture her lying down by the foot of my bed. The odd thing became my mood swings, which gave my husband the incentive to scatter magazine articles encouraging hormone therapy all about the house. When at work or away from the house, I felt fine. It was upon entering my home I became quite irritable and snapped frequently at my husband.

Jann contacted me some weeks later after an intensive meditation, stating she had communicated with Red Cloud, her spirit guide. After she relayed her personal messages she added there was a message for me, but she hadn't a clue to its meaning. Of course feeling childish I never told anyone about my secret pet.

She told me Red Cloud had said to tell Mary to get that wolf spirit out of her house. A wolf spirit is a wild thing and not meant to be brought inside and that it was affecting my temper. He told Jann I needed to make it leave and smudge the entire house. She then added: "I don't know what that message meant, do you?"

I let the wolf out the door that night, the house got smudged and she only gets called back in urgent cases. To add to this, a family member's pet Labrador, a slobbering fool who loves everyone, went berserk one day when I was in the midst of my wolf fantasy. He howled, cried, barked then ran from me, tail between his legs. Everyone laughed wondering why he acted like that. I knew!

A few times during a Sweat Ceremony, I have heard Charles say—"Get that wolf spirit out of here!" And I wonder, does any one ever slide comfortably into this reality?

Around 1990, I also discovered each time I looked up in the sky I would catch a glimpse of a hawk circling. I began to see some synchronicity and asked myself what does the hawk represent to me? Now, most likely since I first noticed this in Florida they were probably turkey buzzards, but none the less, the message came through. When I saw one, I became alerted and began to search out my lesson. I began to notice which direction it flew or circled and thus able to determine what the message meant. The Hawk became my companion and messenger.

I began to notice even my meditations became more influenced by the Native American culture. Once, I remember thinking about Native American names and how they were given, so naturally I wanted to know what name I might be called and moved deeply into a contemplative mode to search. I felt the spirits gather around me and call out: THUNDERBIRD. Well, I thought, that is pretty impressive! I asked if it were do to some special merit and they replied—"*NO! Just your very big mouth! A lot of thunder comes out of it. You have a rough time blending your temperament.*" How kind of "Them" to notice!

Several years later I discovered books explaining the medicine wheel in relation to birth seasons and came to discover my birth time put me into the Thunderbird Clan or Hawk Clan. I was also amazed by the striking correspondence to my nature as found in this book under my new given clan. At the time I was given my Indian name, I hardly knew of the medicine wheel, clans or any such lore that might lend me that insight.

The first time I met Charles on that late summer night. He looked up to the sky and said: " The Hawk is my brother. My spirit guide." Then he said: "THUNDERBIRD—mixing hot and cold. The balance of both." I felt he knew my connections to them both, but at that time I knew little of anything, especially of him or his people.

Charles is a Heyokah Medicine man—the contrary. He works with the Powers of the West. I feel in some way those spirit helpers came for me, years before I had a conscious clue as to which way my life would turn. But they knew and ever so subtly they led me to his door. The hawk and thunderbird's arrival in my life was only a hint of foreshadowing to what was soon to become my strange new allies—The Thunder Beings.

Chapter Four

Jann became fondly known as Two Knives after sporting several daggers off her belt. She heard rumor there were "rattlers" throughout the hills and plains and before we left Illinois begged several hospital physicians for anti venom medicine. They refused, stating she had several hours to make it to a local hospital before suffering any ill effect.

She then took measures in her own hands. At the famous Wall Drugs, she bought a shiny sharp saber length knife that would stand more chance of stabbing her in the knee then impaling a snake. Her second knife came in a give away—a cute little utility knife. She has since replaced it with another sword length weapon that could probably skewer a buffalo. When leaving Charles house one day to gather sage for smudging, he took one look at her attire and fell over laughing. "You just have to pick the sage," he chided, "not stab it to death!"

Jann is the native's darling. She brings continuous merriment and laughter to the group with her antics and stories—the omega wolf—the often times clown.

Her attire alone makes one smile.

When going for her vision this year we made another urgent stop in Wall for vision shoes. I can hardly recall any Native American recounting his need for vision shoes. They were a carry over from Saturday Night Fever and impossible to wear climbing up the mountain, but they were the hit and highlight of the trip as far as humorous memories.

On a spiritual quest the year before, I insisted to Jann that we climb Harney's Peak. It was, after all, where Black Elk received his vision and Black Elk was related to Charles. Jann at that time sported some other odd pair of shoes and a walking stick. Within minutes, she realized this was not going to be a fun excursion. Victor, our Native guide and friend, coaxed Jann by reassuring her she could have a Pepsi and hot dog at the top. We quickly panicked thinking we may not have enough money. Of course when we hit the top a couple hours later and realized how could there be a Pepsi stand up there, it was the best joke the Indians had ever played on white folk. Every year we are reminded and asked if we would care to climb Harney and get a Pepsi.

Chapter Five

Now comes the difficult part—explaining Charles. He is an Oglala Sioux, born on Pine Ridge Reservation in the early nineteen forties. Charles entered this world when the ill effect of the missionary's zeal was still imprinting its dictatorship on the reservation Indian. He was placed in Catholic boarding school on the Rez and, like his peers, forbidden to use his native tongue or religion. It was still common practice to beat the savage out of the native. He ran away several times refusing to submit to the will of the clergy, only to be returned for more abuse. As a grown man he comes full dressed in resentment toward Christianity and its spirited soul saving employees.

When observing the family structure of the Native American it is painful to think that their children over the last century and a half were ripped away from loving arms and shipped to boarding schools out east to Christianize and educate them. Many of those children killed themselves rather then face the loneliness from the forced separation or insane attempts to change their culture. It has been our observation that when there is dysfunction in their family unit due to alcoholism or parents lacking child rearing talents, other family members will take over the rearing, raising and responsibility of the children.

Charles, above all, is a man who aside from his spiritual path as a Medicine Man and career path as an Artist is a caring and nurturing human being. That is what he wishes to be remembered for most. He and his wife have fostered, without financial aid for the most part, several of their families young who were left without parents. These children came from gangs, drugs, and abusive backgrounds. In total, Charles and Hazel have brought around eight children through their doors.

I can only say, since we have seen the before and after on some of these off spring, that I wish I had known Charles and Hazel when mine were little. I would have boarded my two in the hopes they would learn to be a part of all creation and honor every living thing. The foster children of Charles and Hazel are treated as a significant part of the community, not tossed aside as little kids who don't understand, or worse, allowed to become petty tyrants and dictators, sending their adult parents into a frenzy. It is hard to explain, unless one spends time with them. They are happy, well-adjusted and tremendously responsible human beings!

More than Charles healing words or art, those children are his testimony and his legacy. Presently he is raising two young girls full time along with three other children that spend much of their time there. The older boys they raised have moved on but are not far from their hearts. Charles and Hazel have never had children together, but they know how to parent. There is no striking or swearing, The only threat I've heard used is if the children don't mind him they get put out back to sit on a rock! My own children would say—big deal! And to these children it is a big deal.

They are never told to leave the room yet one hardly notices their presence as they blend into all settings. When Charles and his family came to Illinois and lodged with me for a few days, I had six people roaming around the house. I felt more comfortable and at ease with these six than most of my own relatives. It makes one wonder what has been lost in isolating our lifestyles and insisting we need all this space around us. It has nothing to do with the number of people invading our space, rather the size of someone's ego that pushes us to the wall and makes us feel cramped.

At a recent wedding I listened as a table of strangers attempted to out do each other in accomplishments and material benchmarks. It is amazing that most of what comes from our American culture is bragging, while most of what comes from the Native American Culture is silence. They are busy communicating inward with that spirit world—while we reach desperately for that world outside ourselves.

In South Dakota, on nights we spent in our tents, we were always, as Charles put it, with tails. We would have three or four kids piled in with us. Jann and I were bent over with aching sides from all the laughter. To add to the craziness we had one "adult" child always running around in the dark yard late at night trying to scare us—the kid's name was CHARLES. There is a great emphasis this past decade to find the inner child. These people never lost it and in knowing them we have been given the precious gift of ours back.

To see an adult creeping through the yard, awaiting his chance for surprise attack, with some odd ball coyote headed hat on, a painted white face and wrapped in a blanket after all have quietly settled in for the night, won me the official Indian name of "Scared a Lot" or "Screams Daily".

The first summer spent with Charles, Jann and I suffered from sleep deprivation, for when it wasn't the pretend spirit lurking around in the yard, it was the real phantom occurrences that were equally as unsettling. It is difficult for us to let go and believe, as we are always afraid to be made the fool. After years of seeing so much occur at that man's house it finally seems normal, but there was a frustrating period of mental combat over logic, until we last surrendered the need for analytical explanations.

Charles' children are accustomed to this phenomena as part of their everyday life and I no longer attempt to come home and share with my own people what occurs out there for it is met with a thick concrete wall of logic, explanation and disbelief. I feel bad at the missed opportunities to bring back the magic, but each has his own road to walk, and selfishly, I'm glad the one out West isn't very crowded.

I fear our white mentality would try again to overtake, market or monopolize what is left of the Indian spirituality, if they really did believe in those spirit powers! The world presently is filled with plastic shamans trying to imitate the Native Path. It is laughable, the last laugh being on people greedy to snatch the power in hopes of impressing and bedazzling others.

Jann and I have occasionally dressed somewhat eclectic native when visiting Charles, attending ceremonies or Pow wows. Of course Charles and his family are dressed in denim and gym shoes. It is a wonderful lesson for all to dress or look like a minority race and walk out into the white populace and feel the stares and strange looks one receives. I can feel the daggers of racism literally hit me and it doesn't feel nice. But the difference is, I can take off the garments and redress myself in white. They, on the other hand, can't remove the color of their skin.

When visiting Devil's Tower last summer, our little group of travelers stopped at the local souvenir shop on the way out to get refreshments. Jann and I walked around browsing and being greeted with friendly smiles while Charles and his family were watched and given disparaging and unwelcome looks. We thought to ourselves, if they only knew or had within themselves the ability to cure the common cold, much less cancer, diabetes or other diseases such as this human being due to his self sacrifice and belief. And they look down at him, instead.

This past summer Jann and I were so oddly dressed at Crazy Horse Memorial that the other tourists thought, I'm sure, we must be part of some act. I don't feel we missed one person's hard long stare throughout the entire place, including the Natives, but at least Charles and his family could roam and browse and blend in as we Whites are so accustomed to doing. The tourists were too busy pointing there pale little fingers at us, gawking and hopefully wasting film on two white midwestern nurses playing Dances with Fools, or simply call us Laughs a Lot!

Chapter Six

Each time I go to South Dakota or attend a ceremony, I am amazed at how the white man feels this urgent need to talk like Tonto when communicating with the Native Americans. Here we see educated adults wishing to carry on a conversation with an Indian who immediately start to speak with a broken dialect as if they have just landed on American soil or watched a thousand reruns of the Lone Ranger. If I were a Native American, I would probably be inclined to smack them up side the head. I do commend their tolerance of our foolishness.

When one prays, it seems logical that one pray from his heart and speak the words he is familiar with, but instead we have a bunch of parrots trying to repeat the dialect they hear the Natives speak, which sounds, on whites, more like a speech impediment then sincerity.

If I were a medicine person most likely there would be a large decrease in population or increase in frogs. I'm glad to hear the Medicine Man's wife also shares that view. As she often states-The Powers know who and who not to connect with.

But Charles just takes it all in, those that act like Tontos, those that come to him once making a multitude of promises and are never seen again, as well as those who come to take from him a scant amount of knowledge, then run back home and play the plastic shaman.

Like most spiritual paths, there may be a need at times for gentle direction and guidance—the how to's. But the most rigid rules I hear in Native American spirituality are the ones demanded by white people who play Lakota Wannabees and instill all these fearful…"you better do this or that will happen stuff". Middle age yuppies acting like a bunch of kids competing for the teacher's affection, or mimicking a parent's orders. I have full respect for the native teachings and the Medicine Man that does the teaching, but often it is: "Charles said…this or that". Charles, at times, can get a bit testy when re-drilled on all his rules, especially the hundred and one he did not dictate.

There is a spiritual drought upon this land that leaves some desperate for answers and looking for direction. Our need for a quick fix leads us to ease on down the road to the next idealistic philosophy that requires little investment. But the Native American path is not an easy route.

It requires work—often physical. We can't pay someone to do our work, build the sweat lodge, make all the tobacco ties, sit up on mountains enduring the elements to wait—no—cry, for a vision. It is a physical and spiritual road that requires our full participation and endurance.

When Charles visits California, he is often asked to perform a Purification Ceremony. The first one he held contained a mix of new agers eager and ready to play native. They slipped inside his lodge then undressed or unwrapped the towels to be open, free and naked. This might be fine for an all male or female sweat, but this time Charles could be heard three blocks away ranting and raving and stating: "Get those damn clothes back on and show some respect in here!"

Next, he flung a battalion of water bottles out of the lodge, in every direction. The group had wanted to sip on their sport bottles while sweating. There would be no water bottles in Charles' sweat. Besides, the odds were high for plastic melting in one of his purification ceremonies. In most cases, Charles is a great, nurturing teacher, who often jokes. People greatly appreciate this humor as it begins to ease the mounting tension one feels as they start to melt.

Charles, Jann—alias Two Knives, and myself have disagreed on our philosophies at times, but we respect his strength to remain true to his beliefs. I have never seen him sway from his Truth. I am hard pressed to think of many others I can say the same about. Most of us tend to teeter on some fence, jumping off from time to time, when the winds of discordance blow toward us.

But Charles is unconcerned about others' inability to remain steadfast in their convictions. He believes what he believes and there is no fluctuation. But in the same vein when asked who do you answer to, he smiles when you say only to God—Mystery. It is between That and myself.

I think the Heyokah, who is known as the clown—trickster, part of him loves to test! He seems, at times, to fish around inside someone and weed through their fears and insecurities. He coyly baits the hook—then quickly tugs out their insecurities and states: "If it is sickness you fear, you may be ill. If it is loneliness you loathe, it may be your life's calling. If it is love you are seeking, all lovers may have vanished." One is sometimes left open and vulnerable, which allows space for a healing to occur. People can't lay claim to a healing until they know their illness. Charles finds it, and makes a person face it. Once the dysfunction hits the air, it usually goes away. He has a real knack for discovering your shadow, pulling it out and letting it box with you! After all he is Medicine Man and not all cures come in pill form.

Chapter Seven

The first summer Jann and I stayed with Charles we shared a bedroom. Now, he had two available, but in one room, he claimed to keep a soul. We then were privileged to learn about the little Buddhist Monks that stayed with him the past month and were rudely awakened to spirits hovering over their beds in that soul kept bedroom. We politely asked which room they had stayed in. After bribing the children with candy they finally told us.

Neither Jan nor myself were willing to share a room with this soul. Instead we shared a bed with the cliché 'safety in numbers' reinforcing our morale. And, as there is safety in numbers, we had one of Charles foster daughters camp out on the floor in her sleeping bag to guard us. Two women expecting a twelve year old to fight their spirited battles. That is the summer I was named—Scared a Lot!

That was also the year Charles kept up his litany of chicken clacking sounds. But I was more comfortable hearing the clucks than ghostly footsteps down the hall, pots crashing off kitchen counters at three a.m. (only to be discovered tamely on the counter the next morning) and a various assortment of lights being turned on and off each time I would wake up. There could not be that many people making bathroom runs to warrant so much activity.

That year we were also privileged to hear about a new ghostly apparition. Something called 'chunchilas' or as we fondly called it—the Chimichanga Spirit. These self-invited guests seem to show up during the Vision Quests. A little character with red eyes and spiked ridged back, long tail and nails, seem to appear, as told by our Native friends, every so often and terrorize the supporters camping below. Did anyone seriously think we would be foolish enough to venture out in the yard at night after hearing that?

But, as fate would have it, we had a friend whose husband did go up the hill that summer, leaving her alone in her tipi. It was a true test of friendship as we gathered ourselves, Max the dog, our young indigenous friend, along with three flashlights, a mallet and several chocolate candy bars.

To protect oneself from evil forces and assist in purifying one's self the Native Americans take dried prairie sage, ignite it and allow the smoke to wash over the individual. It is called smudging. That evening, we smudged the inside of the tipi, ourselves, the entire exterior of our little habitat and most likely the dog.

Three nurses who have seen the worst that trauma can display, now reduced to wimps, hysterically whispering and terrorized by little scratching noises on tipi walls, all the while our canvas door constantly flapping through the windless night. Little animals (or spirits?) could be heard scurrying about outside. And perhaps a clacking chicken? Unfortunately, we discovered smudging was unsuccessful at removing trickster humans—that is if there were trickster humans out there that night. Of course we were convinced it was Charles causing the ruckus. Well, sort of!

Later that night, we were summoned to the front porch to view the spirits' changing of the guard. At certain times, spirits or energies descend the vision quest hill, while others go up. Out on the deck we waited and quietly talked, all of us looking like we were lined up at a drive in movie. I hardly expected to see a thing, but when I looked down across the front yard it appeared there was a legion of tall shadows marching across the lawn.

I quickly looked at the treetops but they stood still for there was no wind that night. Then in the flash of one second, there appeared a circle of gray ghostly apparitions dancing all around the sweat lodge fire pit. As soon as you blinked an eye, they vanished. It was a sight that brought gasps from our mouths.

"Did you see that?" I really saw it!" We knew we would never be able to explain such things to others but only experience them for ourselves.

That same summer Charles was interviewed by two State Social Workers for his first official foster child placement. We anxiously awaited their arrival. As I mentioned, Charles told his own Truth, never swaying or playing the game. The women arrived and we rushed out to say our hellos and support Charles. As we casually eavesdropped to see how it was going, we heard Charles diving into Native American Philosophy, spirits, his views on Government and Christianity, as well as in depth descriptions of Ceremony. We were sure these women would hardly understand a word he was saying or find him fit to foster.

How foolish we are at times. Of course he was qualified. Was there any doubt?

Certainly not in his mind. We knew his success rate, we feared others may not get the opportunity to see him, but they did see him, whether they believed all of who he was is uncertain, but to see he was genuine was a fact none could deny.

Chapter Eight

I have this wonderful soft top Jeep Wrangler that would look spectacular flying through the Black Hills of South Dakota. It's where Jeeps belong. Unfortunately it is stick shift and Two Knives swore off clutches when she nearly put her dad through the windshield a decade ago. This always left us searching for a car as hers was much too small. The first year we rented a mid size compact that probably required $40 worth of gas round trip, but the physical price was high as it gave us hip displacements and stiff necks.

The following year we borrowed my husband's big old Caddy. We were in seventh heaven with a huge trunk and back seat for taking our gear and room to spare for sleep in its reclining seats. Two days before our return trip to Chicago, I noticed the car's brakes to be dull. We brought it in to Hill City and after I had a mechanic pull apart the brakes and disconnected the anti locks, switching over to manual, we still didn't have much of anything. My guess was the master cylinder. We were pressed for time, already feeling pulled back to our routine life in Chicago and I was leery of strange city dealerships. A real dilemma—what do we do?

I had a little braking ability, but not enough to stop a car of that weight rolling down one of the Black Hill's roads. The mechanic gave us a route to get back on I-90 without the steep ups and down. I knew, except for La Crosse, WI, we would be on flat land all the way home. We planned to take the gamble.

Needless to say, Charles was concerned about our decision. An hour before we left his place there was a horrendous thunderstorm with lightning cracking trees all around us. We saw one huge violet flash hit a tree across the road and as we all screamed, Charles gave a smile and said: "I just got my message. The Thunderbeings will escort you home and protect you." (Sure, Charles!)

We managed to make it through the hills and when at last on I-90 I pointed out to Jann what a thunderhead cloud looked like, as it was along side our car. She smiled stating maybe that was our protection. (Sure, Jann) Within the hour it was dark, turning into night and from that point through the entire trip of eight hundred and fifty miles we followed an incredible display of lightning. Several times the light show became so phenomenal we pulled over to look or took turns driving. The highway stayed dry the entire time and we only found wet streets on side roads where we stopped for gas. The lightning never left our vision.

Each state we entered started a new set of storm fronts that started in the north and moved to the south in front of our windshield. We kept asking ourselves how could this happen? We were driving much faster than a storm front. And since when does a storm front last over eight hundred miles? Even more riveting was the display of lightning. Explosions like the Fourth of July or a combat movie filled the sky. At that moment I knew, from some inner place, we would come to know the Thunderbeings in a most personal kind of way as the year went by.

We came home with these stories and were greeted with skepticism and disbelief. It is hard sometimes to re-orient back into our other world where Jann and I spend most of our lives. No one cares to see the magic—or dance to a new way of thinking. Most feel it best to keep their brain waves slow and even, rather then dance to the Native's Drum!

Chapter Nine

Here we are, two white women, insisting that we see Red Cloud's grave and Wounded Knee. They both sit on the Pine Ridge Reservation, a place of poverty and desolation, with miles of worthless land occasionally speckled with small towns containing unkempt shack homes whose yards are littered with junk cars. Perhaps an occasional gas station or corner store can be seen if you don't blink an eye.

Charles was hardly thrilled to hear about our desire to see the sites on the Rez. He warned us against it, but a Native American friend, who was involved with the AIM (American Indian Movement) group, won out. She wanted us to see the memorial service for the two young people that were killed in the Wounded Knee uprising back in the 70's. Jann took Charles' warning seriously, and for the entire trip out to the reservation I was lectured regularly how we should only stay for a few minutes, then make excuses to leave.

When Jann gets nervous and decides she isn't happy about something, I hear about it over and over and over. It was a very long drive. We followed our friend into the Reservation driving our own car; we knew we had arrived by the lake size potholes in the road. One could lose a car in them. We eventually pulled up to Jumping Bull's house, a lean-to on the prairie. Part of the FBI shootings might have initiated or finished there, I was not sure. The present day movement to free Leonard Peltier stemmed from this mid seventies uprising.

We joined hundreds of people already gathered on a lower shelf of the prairie under an arbor, where the ceremony was about to begin. The people had at last acquired head stones to place on the graves and this memorial service was created to honor, remember and recognize their two fallen friends.

Jann continued her litany of why we should not stay during the long walk down to the arbor. Then she saw him—as she fondly puts it—her Greasy Guy! He was an AIM leader from one of the Southwest States. Jann's dream man was dressed in a red beret with braided hair, of course the usual denims, and a diagonal banner of emblems thrown across his chest. Now, her tune changed tempo: 'Let's stay, we don't want to be rude, we will never get this opportunity again…'

Our Native friend noticed the slack jawed look on Jann and quickly introduced her to 'greasy guy'. I think she conceived that name from a play, hopefully not from her heartthrob's appearance. For the first time in our many year relationship I looked next to my friend and found a mute. Our Native friend told him we were with the Chicago Tribune and would he pose for a picture. Can you just imagine two white women, dressed in our eclectic early Halloween attire, holding a disposable camera representing a major newspaper? I'm sure he couldn't either, but was nice enough to pose. Jann never stopped staring and as I quickly clicked our moment in history, I could visualize her taking the negative and making posters, coffee mugs, watches and wall paper with his face on everything! (He presently decorates her computer screen save.)

We then proceeded by car to the cemetery, behind hundreds who walked holding large AIM banners. As we arrived in the dusty field, sprinkled with head stones, the mood shifted to dark and somber, It became a tearful scene as the deceased woman named Anna Mae was represented by her mother, a small frail little woman dressed in a tattered coat and head scarf. She sat on a folding chair, hunched over and rocking, as someone interpreted her Lakota prayers. Our hearts felt like they were breaking.

When the ceremony finished, our little AIM friend wanted to introduce us all around to her fellow AIM companions. We were tugged to the front lines to meet a particular Native American, name long since forgotten but face forever etched in my memory. He was the head of some Tribal Council. The man was so massive and scary that if I had seen him in the days of old and been taken as his captive, I would have scalped myself! With a face chiseled in stone, which made the Mt. Rushmore guys look warm and cuddly and a cold glaring stare he asked:—Why are you here? I could hardly remember my name much less a complicated answer such as that. There were several whites in attendance, it was my only hope for survival, to my Scared a Lot name mentality. By then, Jann had found her tongue and politely answered him and then we quietly slipped away, hoping to turn invisible.

After Jann had her eyes filled with Greasy we proceeded to Red Cloud Indian School to visit another cemetery in search of Red Cloud's grave. We must have walked up and down the road ten times in search of his gravesite, shaking a million grasshoppers off our bodies, not to mention the dust that coated our skin. It had to be ninety-five plus degrees. The grass hoppers seemed in ecstasy wildly leaping about the barren wasteland. I thought we had taken a wrong turn and ended in hell.

Finally, I stopped and looked at Jann. "I thought Red Cloud was one of your spirit guides," I inquired.

"He is!" She replied.

"Then why the Hell don't you ask him where his grave is?"

She gave a look of dawning on her face, stopped, closed her eyes for a few minutes then walked directly to where he was buried.

Red Cloud was an Oglala Sioux Chief and considered one of the best military strategists in history. He finally surrendered to reservation life, rather than see his people starve. A sad ending for such a magnificent warrior!

At home, I have his photo on my wall. He seemed a very old man at the time it was taken. He stares out at me—dressed in the full regalia of eagle featherhead dress, buckskin and pipe. A kind and compassionate old face, filled with wisdom and love for his people. I somehow feel he was a patient man, especially when now assigned to my good friend for guidance.

That day became a marathon event of mourning and death, for we traveled next to Wounded Knee—another grave site, marking the slaughter of hundreds of innocent people at the close of the 1800's. Children and women were shot as they ran through the fields in terror of the soldiers' firing rifles. It was hot, dry and dusty up on the hill where the memorial stood and at last Jann and I saw the fearsome rattlesnake—a decaying dead one lying close to the gravesites. The land barely appeared fit for slithering reptilians, as evidenced by the snake's demise, much less people.

I contemplated the Gnostic philosophy where the snake represents Wisdom. But this representation of gnosis lies dead. How fitting, for there was none to be found in the mass murdering of these people, not only here but through other past incidents and centuries. Wisdom screeches to an abrupt halt when man seeks personal greed over humane welfare.

We should have heeded Charles' warning, for once one goes forward to seek truth with an open heart and a relentless pursuit to find the honesty, one can be injured by a loss of faith in who and what we thought we represented. These people entered my heart that day and made a home, one that I hope will always be kept open and welcome.

One of the Lakota ceremonies is called the give away. They give to others instead of taking. Jann and I understood the ceremony well that day as we gave our hearts to a people now living with broken dreams and dusty dry land, overrun with leaping grass hoppers, dead promises and decaying snakes. Not a very fair trade off for those once free spirits of the plains who roamed the land with bountiful hunting. The Lakota tribes were one of the last to be rustled to the reservation and their painful memories are still fresh as each generation reminds the next. Many still recall relatives that experienced Wounded Knee.

The Lakotas still carry unhealed wounds of a culture that was stolen. How, I wonder, can some still be willing to share their mysteries and stories with those once bent on seeing them wiped off the face of the earth? Yet, later that evening we sat on their living room floor, laughing at each others stories, while balancing bowls of beef stew and fry bread on TV trays, and I wonder how I ever lived without them or their generous nature. They are always eager to share their gifts and wisdom—and I am forever grateful to be receiver of such gifts.

Chapter Ten

My favorite analogy of the misguided human being is the story Charles tells of the Christmas tree. Why are people like a Christmas tree? First, he states, take a look at the tree. It is beautiful, dazzling and full of color. Now, picture the ornaments as a symbol of one's education. Look at the lights. Imagine they are one's values and the tinsel represents the outward appearance one strives to maintain. But, what's wrong with the tree?

It is DEAD!

It is cut off from its roots and no matter how beautiful it looks, it soon will die. All trees need to remain connected to their roots in order to survive. So do humans need to remain connected to their source—to be deeply rooted in their beliefs and pierce through the illusions of the plastic world.

There is a multitude of white people playing Christmas trees. Jann and I did not have to look very far to view our own tinsel town lifestyles and agree. We had been on a path, in search of our Truth, but still quite enmeshed in our personal plastic worlds.

So, how does one re-connect, I thought? Obviously my withering branches must have stuck out, for I wasn't sure of the answer. I knew the ending, but not the route to get there. The path is not paved in one day, or one summer with the Native American Medicine Man, or is it found quickly like many new age spiritual roads. It requires sincerity and an honest effort to face your shadow and your fears.

Many people cautiously tread so far down the road, then back off because they must give up too much—be it their beliefs or way of life. Instead, they choose an easier path. New Age has been instrumental in regenerating the Old Age religions and beliefs but moved a step beyond and created a structure of easy routes to bliss that appeal to many.

We have become accustomed to the sheep mentality, so easily led. Just turn on the TV and see where our interests lie. The most difficult requirement along the nature based spiritual path is the utmost sincerity to re-connect and become part of the Mystery—and to live as an equal on the earth, not master.

Just changing a word when addressing other living things from it to thou makes a bountiful difference in our behavior. Respect—probably the number one commandment of nature related spirituality.

RESPECT FOR ALL LIVING THINGS!

Charles told Jann and myself that our reconnection initiates in the Sweat Lodge—symbolic of Mother's womb—a re-birthing. This is a turn in the path that most people are hesitant to make. It is one thing to sit and discuss nature and philosophy with a Native American teacher in an air-conditioned hall or living room, but nothing compares to sitting with a Native American teacher who is really giving opportunity for learning by sharing space with him in a Sweat.

Re-connecting, shedding fears, shedding the plastic world, seeing illusions melt away in hissing steam filled huts. Watching, listening and praying—aware of that other world making its entrance into the lodge and your life, and into your soul.

Now, as fate or synchronicity would have it, the 1997 holiday tree for the White House lawn was chosen from South Dakota and Charles was chosen as the recognized Medicine Man of the Cheyenne River Sioux Tribal Council to perform a ceremony at the tree's cutting in South Dakota and lighting in Washington DC.

Here went the man with the Christmas tree story, the man with the warnings about the plastic world heading to Washington to light an unconnected tree in a district that supports acrylic mentality and lifestyles. It was more than coincidence.

He gathered his family and off they went. We thought Washington may never be the same. He stopped in Illinois to greet us, for Charles not only viewed this as a tremendous honor but partial fulfillment of his ancestor Black Elk's Vision. Black Elk had seen those of all nations and colors some day gathered around the flowering tree. Charles had already gone out to bless the tree during its cutting in South Dakota with the Department of Forestry, now he was to perform another prayer ceremony at its installation in Washington.

We anxiously awaited the C-SPAN coverage as we were told Charles would be near Newt Gingrich as part of the South Dakota representation. Native American children also attended the tree lighting and were awaiting their cue to perform a traditional dance. I watched and waited as the snowfall turned to rain.

I kept thinking I must have missed something or tuned in late, for there was no sign of Charles or any Native American. Instead, Senators bellowed out Christmas Carols and children from the Pierre, South Dakota all white choir chimed in. The only mention of an Indian was when Mrs. Gingrich mentioned how the reservation folk were treated to some coats and again when she wished to educate the non Christians in the audience about the meaning of Christmas.

As I watched, my mouth fell wide open. How can this still be going on? I thought, did.... Charles make a mistake? For, at times, I am still too naïve and trusting of a nation that insists it wants to help the misfortunate and treat all with equality.

Charles returned through Illinois and prepared a small ceremony with his family and friends. He lifted his gaze upward and prayed, arms outstretched, to his Lakota Ancestors that—Yes indeed, they still were here, alive and well. We, his friends, stood out there on the front lawn and joined in song, our eyes clouded with tears, while watching this beautiful band of people petition to be honored, heard and recognized.

And it was most likely at that point my Scared a Lot name became Warrior Woman, for in passion and the heat of anger I besieged

Washington with my mighty pen and shouted to all within hearing distance my disdain over the treatment of these people. There comes a point in time when we need to recognize each other as equals and ignore the various colors that coat our bodies. I doubt it will be resolved in my lifetime, but someone needs to wake up and realize where true illusions lie.

Charles performed his ceremony and I began performing. Enough to make Charles realize that perhaps this should be taken as more than another misunderstanding and oversight from his white counterparts.

He took my letter to the Native Council in Minnesota who in turn added their own words of disdain and sent it on with a petition. It resulted in a telephone call from the White House to apologize, but no more than that.

He was promised $800 in traveling expenses. When all was said and done the Forestry Department handed him a few hundred and said that was all that was left.

Charles telephoned after attending the Minnesota Council with kind words and laughter over our attempt to chastise the Capital. We heard the pride, love and friendship he felt for us as he fondly called us Warrior Women and witnessed a softer side of our staunch, tough skinned, hardly approachable Lakota Medicine Man.

And now it was time to discover the man behind the medicine and the friend behind the healer. Jann and I were hook—line and sunk into the Lakota Spiritual Path with the ease that comes from knowing you are walking the right road and following your bliss.

There were still many moments of hell, as following any road has its potholes and bumps, but nonetheless, it was one we chose to freely follow. It didn't matter anymore what others thought or said. This was our way. This was the way our hearts were led, with minds that followed and spirits at last jumping wildly in excitement for their opportunity to at last be heard.

Chapter Eleven

After participating in Sweat Lodge Ceremonies and supporting Vision Quests the next reasonable step was to move forward to the next ceremony. The Sun Dance. The name sounds fairly light and harmless, but it is another form of endurance and sacrifice that the Lakotas, along with other Native Americans, feel is necessary to assist in their spiritual journey and promote a wellness for the whole community.

The ceremony was banned from the Reservation for several decades, yet due to the determination and perseverance of the Plains Indian, it survived, in spite of the clergy's frantic attempts to dissuade or dilute the ritual. The dance is centered around a chosen cotton wood tree, which has been decorated with tobacco ties and ceremony flags filled with the prayers of the people. The sun dancers are presently composed of men and women, although it is the men that usually pierce.

The piercing is a difficult thing to watch, so instead Jann and I would lower our heads and just pray for these people who feel the necessity to take on the suffering of someone for their healing or best interests of the whole.

We have often questioned how many clergy would be left in the ministry if they also were required to sweat and pierce for their congregation. We, as Christians, have adopted spectator participation toward our faith. We allow the man, hanging up there, to—*do it*—over and over again. There is no consideration for personal sacrifice unless one considers opening his pocket book to donate.

The Sun Dancers (men) wear wreaths of sage on their heads and bare chests. They dress in a skirt type wrap of red or white. After a dancer has been pierced he is taken around the circle by a couple of men. If this scene of a man with blood dripping down his bare chest, a wreath wrapped around his forehead and donning red does not symbolically look like something else here, one must be blind to not see the similarity.

Jann and I have come to the conclusion that Jesus was indigenous, for His life seem to duplicate the natural way. He owned nothing, He spent long periods fasting and praying. He definitely appeared nomadic and lived well in a community environment. There are many stories about His gathering with people to share stories; food, laughter, prayer and lastly He pierced Himself—the ultimate sacrifice for His people.

We saw that same thing at the Sun Dance. I could now at last imagine as I walked through the camp, what life must have been like for these people a few hundred years back. Their determination and will kept them alive, while still holding on to the old ways. What an honor to be allowed a living glimpse into the past.

The thought of piercing is far more brutal then the actual event with its supporters singing and the wonderful beat of the drum. It does indeed appear somewhat barbaric in the explanation, especially in our high tech way of life. And most especially to a couple of nurses who have had sterile technique hammered into their brains.

Laying a man down in a dusty field and having men with unwashed hands pierce him with questionable pieces of bone, then rub some strange dry powder into his wound when completed? Not from my civilization have I seen something like that.

Charles is not a Sun Dancer, nor will he ever be. That is a whole different breed of person. It was highly unlikely we would be involved with Sun Dance Ceremonies when in South Dakota, however: we came across another group of Native Americans, in the Midwest, and attended some of their get togethers.

Through this group we were invited to support the Sun Dancers in our own southern part of the state. Jann was not as enthusiastic as I, for she felt the scene of piercing was something she did not care to view. We volunteered ourselves as nurses in first aid, packed up our gear and off we drove to a National Forest. We hadn't a clue of knowing what to expect. Since we were uncertain of the camping situation, we acquired a motel room within five miles of the Sun Dance site that could be compared to the roach motel seen on bug spray advertisements.

Jann had recently watched one of those TV magazine shows that gave a detailed expose on motel hygiene. It was most difficult convincing her to remain there. However when the heat index reached one hundred plus and we found the accommodations at the Sun Dance site on a Neanderthal level, she readily gave in.

The next difficulty came in our volunteering to nurse. We were immediately faced with blisters, ticks, burns, and spider bites, as well as heat exhaustion—things that neither a Critical Care or Hospice nurse had a clue to mend. Next time, we plan to purchase a basic wilderness-training book, or bring along a Boy Scout.

The kitchen facility was a roofed, but open, shelter. There were camp stoves, basins and a hose along with multiple coolers of perishable food. The ice melted at jet speed while people arrived in herd proportions and always hungry. But for the amount of people scattered throughout the camp it always appeared gentle and quiet. The Sun Dance was held further away from the encampment with a separate sleeping area for the participants.

The Ceremony lasts four days. The temperature remained over one hundred degrees for the duration. These brave dancers were without food or water the entire time, with many choosing to participate in the Sweat Lodge nightly.

We could not believe they were alive much less dancing in such intolerable conditions. Their endurance is overwhelming, to we who can hardly endure a flat tire or lack of parking space. We watched them dance and sing and pray and soon joined in, fully entrenched in the sacredness of it all. We know people back home who think sticking needles in their eyes would be more tolerable than some of the adventures Jann and I embark on, but we both feel honored to be allowed to witness such events in our age.

On the other side of the coin, the southern mentality was something to be dealt with as this Indian thing seemed highly suspicious to the town folk. Some suspected that the ceremony might be an orgy or drug fest in disguise.

When Jann could not bear the thought of eating the culinary feast called garbage can stew, a cuisine delight of every vegetable and meat known to man, placed in a brand new garbage can and cooked over the fire for about twenty hours, she and I would venture into town. Her favorite fast food place is Hardys, and of course all little towns have Hardys, so there was a glint of joy in her life.

The thing we overlooked, in our hurry to eat familiar food, was our attire. We would venture into a small fast food place and be stared down by the customers. It was easy to read their minds—we were the enemy. Difference is not cool!

And heaven only knows why Jann felt the need to wear one of her long Reba Red Head wigs to this steamy and torrid part of the country, but she gets these creative urges and feels the need to follow them. One evening we stopped at a local gas station on the way back to our wonderful hell motel as Jann had discovered they sold her favorite drink, the frozen slush cola.

The night had been long, hot and humid. We walked into the tiny store and were greeted by the cashier who was engrossed in deep conversation with a local.

As Jann was busy making her frozen slurp, I immediately noticed her wig was pulling up on her head and therefore making her face look the length of a horse's. I had a difficult time containing myself. She looked at me, puzzled, then caught sight of herself in the window. She let out a howl that would chase away a werewolf and bellowed in laughter that shook the walls. The two locals gave us another of those famous penetrating stares, assured we must be on something, besides exhaustion.

Jann kept repeating she had never looked this bad in her entire life, then fell into fits of laughter again. The customer slowly eased out the door, but not before rolling his eyeballs to the ceiling. Our attire in itself was enough to make one stare. Add a massive red wig on a very long face and it leaves one's mouth gaping wide enough for a Mack truck to enter! Now ask us if we cared?

Between Hardy's and the frozen slush, Jann remained fairly manageable, except when asked to help participate in meal preparation. This, she insisted, she could not do without becoming ill. She even volunteered for hard labor doing the men things, as she put it, before putting one foot in the camp kitchen. Jann, obviously, was not a girl scout.

After taking a year off we plan to attend the Sun Dance this summer. This time we are well equipped with Wilderness Training 101, and a revised first aid kit. Our reservations have been made, at the same motel, our consolation being running water. Again, we are eager to reconnect with old friends and build new memories to keep us warm on cold winter's nights.

Chapter Twelve

It really becomes difficult to distinguish when you are the personal brunt of someone's foolish play when living with people who love to laugh and play jokes. The Native American simplicity is charming, almost child like, except when it comes for our need to know what is real or pretend. Jann and I find it best to believe all odd occurrences at the House of Charles are human produced pranks. It keeps our sanity in check and heart rates steady. However there are some things that continue to roll around in our mind, refusing to settle in as make believe.

Last year Jann and I accomplished a wonderful feat. We purchased a tent and remained inside it the entire week. Charles was impressed! He expected us back in the house by day two, but even through rain and humidity, we, like the U S postal workers, endured. Of course, most of those nights we had our tails with us, making sleeping comparable to a sardine can. All of us, lined up in a row, barely able to take a deep breath. We have a two-room tent, but these little Native children know better. No one volunteered to sleep separately.

On one of those nights, we managed to fall asleep at last, with arms and legs flung all about, six of us sharing a five by five foot space. About three a.m. I awoke to this god awful howling that penetrated the Black Hills from Charles' back yard to Mt. Rushmore. It even overwhelmed the tethered hunting dogs camped next to us who insisted on marathon barking contests.

It was so loud, I could not imagine anyone not hearing it, including our family back in Illinois. All the while, the children continued to sleep. I lay there, absolutely frozen. So terrorized that to breathe was painful. All I could see in the dark were the whites of Jann's eyes as she stared back at me, sheer panic on her face. With a faint little whisper she said: "What was that?" As if I knew!

Then it came again, even louder, and now the big brave hunting dogs outside began to whimper. (The only positive side to this whole episode.) I find it amazing that we didn't wet our pants. All I could imagine as I stared at our paper-thin tent, was that whatever was outside could be inside in a flash.

It sounded bigger then a bear, but then it was probably Charles, wasn't it? And where were those kids when you need them? We waited about ten minutes and when nothing else happened, I find it incredible to believe now, Jann and I unzipped the tent and hurtled through the yard, up the steps and into the house. Our bladder control was losing fast.

Both of us ended up sitting on the living room couch trying to analyze the noise and became increasingly timid about returning to the wilds of Charles' yard. The children remained noiselessly outside, either sleeping or eaten.

To stave off hysteria, we convinced ourselves it was Charles toying with our minds. Then we heard footsteps coming from the level below. Charles entered the room, wiping and rubbing his eyes like a little kid who has just woken up from a deep asleep. He asked us why we were in the house and who made all that noise in and out of the house? We, in turn, kept insisting he confess it was he making that entire growling racket outside, but he never did admit to it.

The next day, I took a poll. I went around to everyone there and asked if they had heard this thing before.

"Of course," they chimed in.

"Well? What is it?" I impatiently waited, tapping my foot.

"Big Foot!" They casually replied, as if it were the local newspaper boy.

"Big Foot? A real...LIVE.... Big Foot?" I gasped.

"Oh no," they would laugh at my silliness, "just a Spirit!". Of course some would smile, winking and I was never sure if the wink meant that it was Charles, or they were just winking. My final conclusion? I don't need to hear that noise again to be convinced-either way!

Chapter Thirteen

There are times when Jann receives inspiration from some unknown source and, like a pit bull, refuses to relinquish this new blossoming thought until it has come to fruition. Last year, one of these ideas kept circling through her brain and thus came to the conclusion that if we wished to spiral ascend toward the true essence of Native American Spirituality, then we (WE??) should make the Vision Quest.

Now, the year before I was very vocal concerning the craziness of any individual doing such a thing. One making a vision quest is denied food and water, made to sweat before going up and sweat after coming down, with the average vision length of time being four days. My Italian nature considered the lapse of time between lunch and dinner a hardly tolerable fast.

Unfortunately I had conveyed these beliefs to my mother, who is still making Novenas of thanksgiving that I had survived the Native American Sweat. I would never be so foolish as to attempt this quest. It was meant for Native Americans and this is one ceremony I would gladly allow them to keep for themselves.

I was also forewarned by my own daughter, who emphasized that my lack of Native background would perhaps induce some paranoia up there as Indians are accustomed to spirits and the likes, unlike our culture who keeps them bound in leather books of supernatural fiction or religion. I knew I would be flying off the mountain at the first sign of any supernatural occurrence, including twigs snapping or leaves crackling in the dark.

My Indian name was Scared a Lot, and with good reason for if I thought death would occur in a sweat, I knew without a doubt, I would be history if I climbed up that hill. The mere thought curdled my blood and left me weak. I was terrorized enough just hanging out at the bottom of the hill these past years while supporting others. A winning Lotto ticket buried up there would not tempt me to go. Only insanity would drive me to it. But then I had to consider Jann's litany, like a thumbnail across the chalk board, insisting hourly that—*We need to do this, It won't be that bad, You need to think about it too, This will be a good thing.*

Unless a lifetime on Prozac was a good thing, I could not imagine coming through this well balanced and happy.

Just the thought of it made my legs buckle and left me convinced it was time we started down separate paths. She would walk up and I would stay down and support her. We had endured several sweats that year. I was actually beginning to feel good about my endurance capabilities and a little remiss at not having access to Purification ceremonies back in Illinois. However, I still held some fear at being attacked by a "gourd spirit" while encased in blackness and sweating profusely. Now, if one can imagine this grown woman Velcro'd to the back of the lodge wall in avoidance of a being whacked by a rattle, one can see why going up a hill, all alone, in the dark would be absolutely inconceivable. And more daunting was the apparent lack of fear Jann displayed at going up.

I knew about two Lakota words. Tatanka (buffalo) and Tankashilah (Grandfather) The spirits and I would have a most difficult time communicating up there—so, why bother them? I could mimic some of the songs in the sweat, at whisper level when the lodge was full of loud voices, but to attempt to sing a Lakota song by myself? Ridiculous! To even think of learning the language in one year—not in this old brain!

Jann left Charles that year committed to making a vision the following summer. I left there undecided, mostly, to even continue on a path that required absolutely too much of me. Wasn't sleeping outside in the rain with Big Foot growling enough bravery? And what about all those Sweats I had endured, actually enjoyed? What more could these people want from me, this middle aged white fluff? My style of "roughing it" was a Motel 6, for God's sake. Was it worth losing my sanity over? I was convinced I would return from that mountain forever banished in some mental ozone.

But that was the year the Thunderbeings escorted us home, and it was on the way home, I knew, no matter how much I cried, complained, whined and bellowed, that my spirit would be dragging my body up that hill, no matter how hard I fought.

Jann and I came home and fell instantaneously into a black hole. I think the gates of hell opened up and sucked both of us through, into a parallel world for all people and situations seem to turn into one huge festering difficulty.

Jann kept commenting throughout most of that year that she was in some void, feeling nothing, doing nothing. All spirit guides had vanished and we seemed to be wandering aimlessly through our lives and year under some huge cosmic test. Egos were attacked, yanked out in front of us to view and then under the mortar fire of our friends—they were blown up!

Spiritual preparation? Hardly! Survival of one's sanity as we tossed fragile egg shell ideas back and forth as how to prepare at all for such an undertaking. I, who organize my date book on a daily basis, had a most difficult time trying to organize this venture. I even found a book on how to "do" a Vision Quest. But that didn't prepare me. How could it? Visions are personal endeavors. One can't take others lessons to educate themselves.

Often during late night sessions, Jann and I tapped out all fears, objections, conclusions and doubts across our Internet e-mail. One minute I would attempt to lift her spirits, the next moment, I would chastise her foolishness to even consider such a crazy thing. She in turn kept plodding along, no matter what I came up with to terrorize her about this foolish Vision.

She knew, no matter what, we would both be up on that hill next summer. I became a master at concocting every excuse known to humanity and developed good reasons to stay down.

There were a few requirements asked of us by Charles to make our Vision the traditional way. I wasn't some darn Indian, I retorted angrily one night to Jann. How were we going to gather these requirements? Why should we, anyway? Isn't there any mercy for us whites making this Vision? Feathers, and abalone shells? Making six hundred and six tobacco ties? Stakes from a willow tree? I could hardly tell an oak from a maple!

And this same daughter of mine, who said—"Ma, don't do it!" Now became a sage and sat back relaxed and assured all would be fine and work out perfectly. Was the whole world going crazy? This is me—Scared a Lot, remember? I could hardly tell my own mother about this crazy plan, for fear it would hospitalize her to know her supposedly grown up daughter was living out childhood adventures by climbing up some Native American's Black Hill eager to dehydrate and starve herself senseless for the sake of what? What was the reason, I again asked for the thousandth time?

Besides, I wouldn't recognize a Native American vision if it slapped me in the face. I have visions! White visions, in nice soft beds with meditation tapes playing in my ears. I have, over the years, received wonderful visions. Why go for one more?

This also became my bone of contention with Jann. She wanted a vision. I wanted my life! Through all this childish meandering, the one focal point that kept surfacing was my fear of just being outdoors, alone, at night. I was a Girl Scout once, who relished the outdoors and adventure. I thought camping was a bit of heaven. At times, after reviewing my childhood memories, I even compared myself to Marlon Perkins, catching snakes, frogs and turtles. Every week mother had to remove these creatures from her stationary tub to do the laundry. I lived in cowboy boots during my teen years and learned to ride horses before school age. Why was the thought of this so difficult? Where had I lost myself, taken a wrong turn and become someone so strange and foreign to nature that it had became comparable to a personal experience of living horror on Elm Street.

The winter came and so did Charles as he passed through to Washington to light the Holiday Tree. Funny! It was me that pushed Jann one afternoon to give him the tobacco required to make our petition for a vision official. Why? I knew there came a time when we would be asked to get off his living room floor, one where we felt such comfort and peace, in the midst of laughter and story telling, and make the commitment. To honor these people and their ways, I felt I must at last show my respect for them and their beliefs. To 'walk my talk' as one says.

Yes, God willing, the Great Mystery Willing, we would go up on that hill for I knew deep inside, I would go no further, nor would Jann till we ascended up! Somehow, as crazy as it sounds, we each felt observed by unseen eyes. A test, so to speak. Without grades or awards that would credit this adventure by human measurements. Another benchmark not meant to score a pass or fail, rather just another human experience in the so-called school of life. Would we really become those Human Beings that Charles so often mentions and misses? We would give it our best shot!

And besides, I was sick of the name Scared a Lot! But, I still planned with great caution to make some effort to control my strange and foreign environment. Like—sneaking up my buck knife. And, perhaps a cellular phone—just in case?

Chapter Fourteen

At some point during our year of preparation, I knew, just absolutely knew from the bottom of my shoes, we would be questing during a thunderstorm. I kept visualizing this lightening flashing all around me. Enough to make me forewarn my friend and secure a rain poncho and plastic table clothe as covering.

The message drifted in to my conscious at some point between the bolts of lightning and cracking thunder we were graced heavily with last spring. But, I thought, the good news was that Charles would be up to instantaneously rescue us, if indeed that should happen.

I knew he had to retrieve his wife one year due to severe weather conditions. Could I not stand a few moments of clashing lights and booming thunder, if it meant bypassing an entire night on that mountain? Of course!

I now can laugh at my ignorance of this whole situation.

I should have realized that our Medicine Man works with the Thunderbeings and they are the ones that bring the vision. I hardly understood the sacredness of the whole event and of course misjudged the power of prayer as I had Two Knives praying desperately for a Vision. Not to mention, the traveling Thunderbeings who took us home one year were sure to bring us back the next.

Two Knives was getting the message not to bring much up on the hill, as she was meant to experience discomfort while I, on the other hand, was packing a vision bag! Could anyone be more white then that? I was paralyzed with fear, to the point of not only questioning my sanity but tossing out a few sketchy last minute bequests in the event of an untimely death. Jann seemed in some ways unapproachable. I could not persuade her to reconsider and I now felt my own personal tugs toward the mountain leaving me no choice but attempt the vision or feel ashamed of my fearful nature for about the next five lifetimes.

I considered perhaps having an accident, or be out of commission with a menstrual cycle, as that puts an end to any form of ceremony. But all of us, our supporters included, just knew both of us would be up on that hill. I could feel destiny pulling me, by her teeth.

Of all years to start my menopausal complaints, I was convinced I fell into hell. I ran through hot flashes, hot tempers and hot language. I went on and off hormones and in and out of various bodywork sessions. It was in some odd way a preparation, all on its own. We originally intended to fast routinely, each time extending the length. We thought of bringing journals, leaving them behind, learning Lakota songs, learning Beatle tunes, as I was assured the major theme song sung by our fellow spirit teachers was Fools on the Hill.

Do we take music or meditation tapes? Do we remain traditional and take only the Pipe? What does one do all those moments, alone, after praying?

White and Red, now running through our veins, a swirling of both worlds, making us stand out like barber's poles, rather then well adjusted Human Beings.

As time for departure grew nearer, my nerves grew thin. I knew I would never again challenge myself in this way, in this lifetime. It had to be done and it had to be done right!

Chapter Fifteen

Mitakuye Oyasin—a Lakota phrase meaning we are all related. But the relationship goes beyond human, into the animal and plant kingdom, the rocks, the stars, sun and moon. It was my hope to have a reunion with my long lost relatives, those that I considered non living or insignificant a decade ago. Now, the hawk became my messenger, the stones in the Sweat Lodge bore faces and Thunderbeings spoke in some unknown but understood form of communication.

We arrived in South Dakota with our supporters that year—three young woman of thirty, who were eager to share our vision and the Medicine Man's ceremonies. Another good friend volunteered to cook and was thus referred to as Warrior Beef Stew Woman. She did not come to seek out a new faith, as she was content to remain in her own Christian faith. Rather, she came as a friend to encourage us on our quest and full respect was given to her beliefs. Charles, in fact, was so delighted with her culinary feats that he told her to stay out of his sweat as it may lessen her ability to cook. This was unheard of, from Charles.

We spent the first few days in South Dakota adjusting to the reality of the Vision's proximity in our lives. We ventured into the task of making our tobacco ties, as well as sharing in the Vision Quest stories of those who had just come off the mountain. We spent time with Charles and his family waiting our day up on the hill, our stomachs knotted, yet spirits eager to move forward through the next unknown door. I immediately asked Charles about the weather. Has it been raining, as in thunderstorms? No, he replied, it has been nice. Wait, I thought.

The kids helped us make ties into the late hours of the night, our laughter at their antics bellowing throughout the halls and hills. And, as time drew nearer these children with full sincerity pledged to fast with us in support. Jann and I could not believe their willingness to do such a thing. A group of twelve and thirteen year olds, choosing to support and take part in our quest. No higher honor could be bestowed than the sincerity and intentions spawned by youth. Now, when Jann and I look at their ties wrapped neatly around our altars, filled with the prayers of these innocents, we will have the strength to endure anything, I'm sure.

We didn't have to wait long for our new other world friends to arrive for as we finished the very last of our ties, the thunder, rain and hail moved in to say hello. It was beginning. Our fast began at midnight that night. I had brought a movie camera along to capture the carefree moments. Now, looking back one could, instead, easily witness the lines of stress etched deep into our expressionless faces, framed forever—the final tormenting hours.

The next morning, we woke up and then we waited—both of us quietly gathering our thoughts and things—for when in South Dakota the time changes to Indian time, something that can't be calculated, just patiently endured.

At last the Sweat Ceremony began. In mid afternoon, the Thunderbeings rolled in to watch and Charles became anxious to get us up on the hill for their arrival was his sign. Yet, he did not hasten the ceremony nor lessen the endurance. His regular singer/ drummer was ill therefore leaving him to call in the spirits with an old ancient song that left everyone still as the melody struck deep within each soul.

Outside the rumblings continued. Jann and I feeling panicked momentarily that perhaps we are much too ignorant to be in the midst of all this power so neatly contained and packaged in this place, man and culture. We were allowed some water during the sweat ceremony. Aside from that I remained without solid or liquids for forty hours, while Jann endured about fifty two. The physicians back home threatened and warned such foolishness would most definitely harm us, but I could hardly recall one long moment where weakness overcame me, or thirst and hunger.

Have we forgotten completely any form of endurance? People of retirement age, climb that mountain, without as much as a whimper or complaint. We have allowed technology minds to rear and control us. Before I began this vision, I also could not comprehend a lack of food or water, with sweats and intolerable heat added. But, it happened, with hardly a notice of discomfort.

Jann and I were taken up to the top of the hill, the clouds quickly rolled in and the final prayers were murmured. Tied into our altar, although not literally, we were told repeatedly how safe we were—if we remained inside of it. Nothing can harm us within the altar.

Nothing! That night was my true test of faith as the lightening struck all around the pine forest The thunder instantly following as I lay huddled under my plastic cloth, my whole being dampened and drained, yet there was a feeling of being held in a safe place. Others who had braved that hill told me that I would know and understand and receive my lessons and directions. But from who, I thought and how? But the messages came through the entire night, gentle and encouraging, as if talking to a child.

At first I was naïve enough to think Charles would dash up the hill and rescue us, but the only thing that came to greet us was more rain and thunder. As darkness closed in, I heard a drum beat from below and was thankful someone thought to play and cheer us on. The beat was different than I had heard before. It made me want to rise and dance as it resonated somewhere deep in my soul. I made mental note to ask which song accompanied such rhythm, as I could not hear any voices. Later, I discovered there was no one playing the drums that night, at least not human. It was the drumming, Charles explained, that accompanied the spirits who rise up to meet the Vision Quest seekers and its beat is the natural rhythm of Mother Earth.

There are times I long to hear her heart beat again and this time dance to her rhythmic tune. There are times I wish others could hear her beat and know the magic that I have experienced. I heard the drum beat and it was like no other—and gratitude is the only word I can think to say.

Before darkness came I made my round of prayers to the six directions. I could occasionally catch a glimpse of Jann, further down the hill. She appeared all right, about as all right as I was. My sincerest prayer was to be left undisturbed by spirits or spooked by noises as the storm was enough to test my courage and sanity. They heard my prayers and forest creatures know best not to venture out on stormy nights, unlike their two legged counterparts.

While we were enduring the elements and praying on the hill, my daughter and friends slept in the house below and were gifted with their own lessons of courage. They had spent late hours out on the porch, plastic garbage bags over their heads due to the rain, but watching a multitude of lights come through the yard, weave in and out of Jann's and my tent, then move up the mountain.

The lights came in intervals during the night, as if taking shift watch. When the next set arrived the other lights came down the hill passing each other along the way. It is hardly something one can describe or scientifically explain, except to picture lots of Tinker Bells floating around in various sizes and colors. It was enough to convince all who remained below the sacredness and power of the Vision.

When at last the supporters moved inside and quietly settled on the living room floor, these same young women were terrorized by growling spirits, that Charles later explained as bear medicine. "Because it growled", he chastised their fearfulness, "you thought it a bad thing, instead of a good sign. It came to bring you a message and you scared it away." How can one rationalize or explain such occurrences? And with that—I say no more.

I came down the next morning, cold and shaking. At some point during the night, I prayed to see the stars, for unless you have seen the endless star filled skies of South Dakota, you can not understand how important that petition be.

After begging for just one glimpse of a star, I was given a view of the Morning Star as she hung like an ornament out of the eastern sky. I don't know how I saw her with all the clouds still hovering, but she was there, as my messenger, to let me know it was finished—my time was over. This time—but now as assured as I was before to never having a next time, I now knew I would be back.

I left the mountain, aware of how much more there is to know and see beyond our limited perceptions. I marched off that hill aware of new concepts and truths, but tucking them securely deep in my soul, for it is my truth and experience. I walked proudly and confident off that hill, yet humbled by the Power and forever grateful of those moments shared in another world.

Getting back to the house, I quickly showered, now welcoming the steam and heat, then found my sleeping bag and nestled in (where else?) but between all the children still quietly asleep. At one point during my rest I felt a presence hover over me and looked back to see the Medicine Man quietly tucking me in. It was a moment I will always cherish for its message to me was one of welcoming me back and recognition that although I had not received a traditional Native Vision, I had attempted to walk down their road, and succeeded.

Jann remained another night up there on that mountain, a test of stamina and determination hardly associated with a Midwestern white nurse embraced in a soft life. She tromped off that hill like Hannibal, with as much strength as when she ascended.

While she lay quietly in her tent awaiting her Vision Sweat, I walked out on the back porch and instantly sensed a deer spirit. I looked at the dog, who seemed oblivious to any intrusion, then within minutes I caught sight of her, before the dog sensed her presence. Twigs cracked as she broke through the brush, the dog at last barking and it was then I knew I had momentarily connected to all living things and was overtaken by the beauty of that connection. Meanwhile, Jann lay out in our tent, fanned by large windy breezes flapping out the tent walls, keeping her cool and comfortable during her last round of endurance. There were no obvious breezes that morning, as we later insisted to her disbelief. Nature held both our hands that day and walked us ever so gently into a new world of love, life and thought.

We came off that mountain, leaving fear behind and newly equipped with energy and inspiration like never before. Although neither of us consciously recalls a vision, something of magnificent proportions occurred to both of us up on that hill, as if we both were instilled with some drive that continues to thrive at the deepest level of our being today. We surrendered to a force higher than ourselves as we climbed up that hill, at serious risk, to return with a better concept and understanding of the Great Mystery.

There are no Tinker bells dancing around man made altars, nor are there growling bear spirits in family's living rooms. There are no mysterious gourds whacking me in my bed at night, nor flicking Bic lights hovering around my steamy showers. There are no extra voices singing in ceremonies, nor flapping, invisible wings hovering over my head, like there are in that Lodge. And, there is no place in that world for analytical minds, nor lack of faith and trust. It just is the way it is! I don't find reason to investigate, explore, justify or explain, rather now just accept the power as it comes in and works with all willing to be open to it.

It is a place that has stood still and remained open to one culture who through trials and tribulations and overwhelming odds chose to remain connected to the power, while our dominant advancing society covered and coated over the Mystery with a new set of scientific values, so that we can hardly see, much less understand or accept any of this as reality. Unfortunate for our culture, now gifted with the best technology in the world but deeply impoverished in faith by that same gift—a double edged sword that cuts and wounds the human spirit..

This could have been where I ended, but more lessons came our way that summer, for now we would be witness to a phenomenal healing, not occurring at Mayo or the best of University Hospitals, but in a Sweat Lodge in someone's back yard—requested by a young woman who chose to push away from conventional and instead summon Charles for a healing—her only payment being her faith and simple tobacco. He heard her plea, gathered his items and family, all piling into his Van, and headed to Chicago within two days notice.

Can you see your doctor doing the same?

Chapter Sixteen

In this final chapter I came to title the book: *Love, Miracles and Medicine Men* as an accessory to Bernie Siegel's inspiring book for people with life threatening illnesses. There is life beyond the conventional and traditional world of medicine. This is a fact I have always been sure of, yet the concrete evidence has sometimes escaped my vision. I have been witness to mini-medical phenomena, actually participated in these events, while channeling Reiki—but a big booming miracle has only been made clear to me after the fact. I wished to see one, for I am in some ways a twin to the doubting Thomas.

Jann and I have witnessed phenomena in the Sweat Lodge but to partake in a healing of this proportion gives one opportunity to at last scream from the roof tops—YES! See, it IS true! Don't listen to my words or believe me. Look for yourself!

The baseline here is—I am white and entrenched for eighteen years in the medical profession, as is Jann but lately, she and I appear as fish out of water in the conservative and traditional hospital setting. I'm sure administration agrees and has wind of our peculiar adventures and I am convinced enough conversations have rocketed through the Hospital grapevine, especially since our return from the Vision, to make most fellow employees very aware of our alternative beliefs.

Occasionally physicians are pulled into these discussions, some filled with humor, others open while still some retort in mocking humor. But at least more are willing to listen, not that by any means should they be encouraged to change professions and jump around their patients drumming in buck skins, but take an open minded approach to their patients. For their lack of faith and disapproval of alternative/complementary modalities is clear on subliminal levels, even when they nod the go ahead to those desperate to live.

It is said one's fate is determined within the first fifteen seconds of receiving a diagnosis. How that doctor conveys the message can carry a life or death sentence.

We can always assume the predictable course in life threatening diseases, but no one knows with absolute certainty. Yet Doctors give time limits, thus squelching the patient's will to accept life beyond that scope of time.

Jann and I hold firm to the belief in honesty, but add to that compassion and the true belief that nothing can be certain. As long as there is one breath left in the human body, there is always hope—not the false type—that some MD's feel a need to present by continuous instillation of poisonous toxic chemo in bodies so weak and ravaged and clinging to their last breath.

But, there is space—wide and open—between the two worlds of healing. The physical and spiritual. We may not always have a cure, but there is never anyone denied a healing and perhaps in some cases death may be the ultimate healing. We can't judge the final outcome as good or bad. It happens the way it was meant to happen. From what we have read, explored and experienced, it is apparent that there is a connection between body mind. There is a connection between energy and maintaining wellness. All disease starts in spirit before presenting and manifesting in the physical.

Taking this as fact, it is easy to observe the Medicine Man/ Shaman's role, for not only is he in touch with the powers to heal, the main healing lies in the spirit/soul. Our modern society, eager to grab on to this new and profound direction that has only been around and used by indigenous people for several hundred millennium, know it has something to do with soul retrieval.

So, now we enter Psychologist's and counselor's offices and see them heavily engrossed with their drums, banging away, and performing various rituals picked out of some book, with their own spice added—to retrieve ones lost soul—and stimulate a spontaneous healing. Hardly ever does anything happen, for it is not a four step process but a way of life.

This is not to say the Medicine Men hold sole stock in the Mystery and Power, but rather instead, have remained connected to this force, where we, as the dominant society, may spend the next several lifetimes unlearning all the damage, before venturing into true alternative/ real healing situations. It does not come from a book, especially the ones written in the English or Middle European languages.

When the industrial revolution entered our realm and technology made advancements in leap and bounds, we put the Shaman into the category of superstition and mumbo jumbo. But, it is time to come back full circle and see the truth that lay before our eyes.

The medical profession is worried, as it is difficult to legislate and license an indigenous Medicine Man. Therefore, some feel a need to diminish and disprove any form of alternative/ complementary modality. It may cut into their power and pocket books, they fear. But where does this leave the patient while sides are taken and lines drawn for battle?

One young woman, exasperated by modern medicine's inability to cure the sarcoma she had been riddled with for eight years, came to a friend one night to ponder different choices. She had heard about Charles and learned of healings he had been instrumental in. But don't we all sit back and say—Well, that was then, but mine is different? This time, frustrated with having to go another round of chemotherapy as the tumors reoccurred within her abdomen, she made the fateful call—what was there to lose?

Charles was at her side by the third day. They spent long hours, at first discussing her faith and present state of mind. He took time to move deep within and discover her belief system. She exchanged tears and laughter, all the while suffering physical pain, which forced her to take medication. But, she stayed open and honest and willing to put her doubts aside and surrender to the Mystery.

The second night, we all gathered on the patio for a Pipe Healing Ceremony. Four of us who had recently visioned shared our stories and offered her words of encouragement regarding the new wave of power and belief. This young woman sat there wide-eyed and listening as we encouraged her to move deep within and find her truth.

Charles had been advised by his spirit realm powers to have a healing Sweat the following night. He never makes plans, but listens and follows instructions from that higher Power. The young woman was given full instruction on what to do and bring, as the only thing required is the post ceremony meal. This was a difficult chore, as she was overcome with bouts of nausea much of the time.

She left us that night smiling but in obvious pain, moving slowly and deliberately. She was instructed to stop all further medication. This would be the most difficult part, she thought.

Although, this is only through hearsay, but from most reliable of sources of friends who attended, the Healing Sweat was like none ever witnessed before. Each Healing, Charles assured me later, is different. This one could be compared, as one friend said, to an exorcism. The young woman was ill before entering due to severe abdominal pain and nausea. Once inside the hot hissing lodge, she felt intense pain, causing her to moan and cry. Twice, she had to leave the lodge to vomit. A nurse followed her outside, per Charles instructions, to give her support and was asked to place her hand on the young woman's belly. The nurse likened the feeling to placing her fingers on a bag of snakes. The woman's belly rocked and rolled as if an alien were ready to pierce through. The nurse became more than alarmed but held strong to her faith in Charles.

The young woman refused to surrender to the illness and twice crawled back inside the lodge, while others prayed in earnest for her healing. Those that attended were amazed as they explained their version of what happened.

The Healing Sweat, at last completed, the young woman finished her evening suddenly feeling famished and attacked her food with a vengeance. All were amazed as a few hours before she was forced to the outside porch when food smells nauseated her. Afterwards, her husband said she slept the entire way home, approximately two hours drive.

His story continued—As he fell into bed until the late hours of the morning, a wife now jumping around their home power cleaning awakened him. She then proceeded to do the laundry, shop, and finally cook a large meal for our group that night. She whistled by him several times as he gazed back in astonishment. The young woman continued to cook, clean, and then serve us, all the while chattering up a storm. She had not taken any form of medication and felt wonderful. She then left us with kisses and hugs to join her husband at a band job. I was exhausted just watching her.

We were amazed to see the once pain riddled, slow moving woman, now almost prancing around with fits of giggles, her voice booming and sturdy.

And we, as nurses, held our breath, for our whiteness and profession will never leave us entirely free on an instant's notice to accept without doubt what we were witnessing, without some other explanation. I held my breath, not that I ever doubted the fact of a miracle, but I was never so privileged to directly witness such an event.

Charles became stern when I held back my enthusiasm, questioning if I were slipping back into that plastic world. But, if that were my only interest, would I have sought him out to begin with? Would I keep returning, in spite of all my fears, to this strange and foreign place?

Would I battle with doctors at the hospital, when their cynicism leaves me cold? Would I have taught my children and brought my children out before this man and encouraged them in this way if I were made of acrylic? And mostly, would I feel this loneliness, returning now to a strange and foreign land that once was my home and comfort?

My enthusiasm was dampened by fear of the failure I had experienced with my brother. I knew then that there is some power that does and can heal. Now, I saw it happen with my own eyes.

It was another beautiful summer evening the final night we again collected on the patio. New faces came through the door. They were friends of the newly healed woman and, like before, an empty chair stood next to Charles. As the young woman approached, he waved her to sit down, with the flag of his hand.

She giggled nervously as she responded to his line of questions. We saw it coming as his eyes, like the hawk, began to focus and take in his next spiritual prey and we knew it was time to get up and leave them alone. When we rejoined them a few moments later, the tissues were out; her head was shaking as tears streamed down the young woman's face. "I don't know how he pulled things out of me that no one knows." She blew her nose, as we all nodded in unison.

" Yes, he has that uncanny quality about him," Jann softly chimed in and offered her a smile.

The young woman with cancer has returned from her doctors with CAT scans that are baffling the medical mind. Her tumors are gone. She has been pain free, full of energy and returned to work. She has not taken one pill. She has moved beyond any placebo affect, I'm sure. The doctor flatly told her this occurrence is not due to the recent chemo injection. It would not have worked that soon nor was it that powerful.

"I am no Holy Man," Charles always will say. "I'd be lying if I told you I am. I'm no savior, nor do I want to be. The healing occurs between you and the Powers, not me. I just bring them here. It's up to you and them. Do you believe?"

The young woman told her doctor where she had been and he just smiled, not in the cynical way, but gently and without judgment. He needs time, he told her, to confer with her other doctors. He is stumped! She is now the one smiling!

That same week, Kate beseeched the Medicine Man with her own need for healing. She approached Charles with the traditional tobacco and asked if he might pray for her dad who was in the advanced stages of disease due to alcoholism.

She and her brother, as well as several other family members had attempted, without success, to come to terms with his impending fate. All previous attempts at encouragement and soliciting him to break free of the disease had failed. She cautiously leaned over toward Charles and placed the tobacco in front of him. She was not looking to cure her dad, rather that he find some peace of mind which would allow his soul to be free before he left this world.

Charles closed his eyes and quietly assessed the situation. He told her that her dad was very ill and then counseled her on letting go. They both sat there quietly and prayed for her dad. She had tears streaming down her face. He gave her instructions on how to ask the powers for help. She came to me the next day asking me to partake in the ritual and added her own when she wrote her father a heartfelt letter of her love to him.

Three weeks later, on her birthday, her father called. He had gone under doctor's care and ceased consuming alcohol. Five weeks later he had lost weight, his blood pressure was normal and his liver enzyme count remarkably decreased. He had no idea what his daughter had done.

Since that time, he has slipped back but again has gone through detox and at last is out of denial that he has a drinking problem. A miracle in itself and the first step in the hard road to recovery. A simple prayer? A child's love? A matter of faith? All had been tried before. This time someone listened! Who?

MIRACLES—It is now a valid word in my vocabulary, and one that both these people, as well as those who love them will add to their list. A man given the opportunity to live again. A young woman restored to wellness. Enough time to allow each the ability to seek new lifestyles and choices for wholeness. How long? Who knows? Will everyone believe? Doubtful! But think of all the energy required to suppress and not believe. To maintain those worn out thought perceptions, because it's much too scary to go to the edge, trust and free fall and eventually land in one's own truth, free of the puppeteer's strings that bind us to small staged dramas of hopelessness in the world of the collective conscious.

A wonderful Buddhist phrase—Better to live one year as a tiger than one hundred as a sheep.

The final leap of faith, an overused phrase in a society paralyzed to make the jump. Dare we be considered foolish or not melded in the mainstream? Dare we sit and sing with Indians, or pray and hold hands with the homeless or hug the crack baby? It may trigger discomfort and thus pierce our stable and sound perception of how we thought the world to be. Instead we may see the space we really inhabit. Or perhaps it's safer to stay apart, unconnected—A Christmas Tree for all to gaze upon and view—See the Beauty?

At least for a short while. Till the branches wilt and lights grow dim.

THE BEGINNING!

Epilogue

March 2000

This book, in manuscript form, sat on my shelf and collected dust for over one year as I was fed up receiving rejection letters and my ego was bruised and battered.. Recently Charles telephoned to say he saw my face on a book that fell from the shelf. We pondered over its meaning and I mentioned this story I had written. He decided I should not give up and he would lay it on top his sweat lodge during the next ceremony. Seven days later I found the resources to have it published.

Peace and Love

Mary (SAGE5001 @AOL.com)

Jann (TWO KNIVES4 @AOL.com)

About the Author

Mary Keiser

Mary Ruehl-Keiser resides in Illinois with her husband Don and their four children- Karie, Kate, Michael and Todd. Her primary vocation is in the healing profession as a nurse, massage therapist and Reiki practitioner. She also writes articles for various Native American web sites concerning Indigenous healing.

9 780595 009732